Y0-AAT-475

THE GOLDEN
HANDICAP:
A SPIRITUAL QUEST

THE GOLDEN HANDICAP:

A SPIRITUAL QUEST

A Polio Victim Asks, "Why?"
And Turns His Life Around

By Garrett Oppenheim, Ph.D.
With Gwen Oppenheim

A.R.E. Press • Virginia Beach • Virginia

Copyright © 1993
by Garrett Oppenheim

1st Printing, July 1993

Printed in the U.S.A.

All rights reserved. No part of this book may be reproduced or
transmitted in any form or by any means, electronic or mechanical, including photocopying, recording or by any information
storage and retrieval system, without permission in writing from
the Publisher.

A.R.E. Press
Sixty-Eighth & Atlantic Avenue
P.O. Box 656
Virginia Beach, VA 23451-0656

Edgar Cayce Readings © 1971 by the Edgar Cayce Foundation.
All rights reserved.
Reprinted by Permission

Library of Congress Cataloging-in-Publication Data
Oppenheim, Garrett, date.
    The golden handicap : a spiritual quest : a polio victim asks,
"Why?" and turns his life around / by Garrett Oppenheim with Gwen
Oppenheim.
        p. cm.
    ISBN 0-87604-306-6
    1. Oppenheim, Garrett, date.   2. Association for Research and En-
lightenment—Biography.   3. Poliomyelitis—Patients—United
States—Biography.   4. Reincarnation therapy—Case studies.   I.
Oppenheim, Gwen, date.   II. Title.
    BP605.A77O66 1993
    248.8'6'-dc20   93-4205

Cover design by Sally Brown

This Book Is Dedicated
to the Memory of My Parents
Whom I Have Finally
Learned to Appreciate

CONTENTS

PREFACE

You may find this book different from most personal accounts you have read in that the author is conspicuously handicapped, a professional writer and a longtime psychotherapist who can, one hopes, communicate in understandable language about the dynamics of a handicapped person. It will go into friendships, therapies, relations on the job, the author's family relations, and his relations to a Higher Creativity, however it manifested itself to him.

Because of the structure of this story, it will proceed more by subject matter than by strict chronology; so please forgive me for skipping back and forth and around within the time frame of my life. This is not an autobiography; it is not an account of one man's conquest of a handicap. Rather, it is the story of my quest for the meaning of a life negotiated with a very visible disability. I have omitted many important events in my life, simply because they do not seem directly relevant to the theme of this book.

I was stricken with polio at the age of fourteen months, and it has been a central fact of my life ever since. It has been both a hardship and a gift, as I will try to explain in the pages of this book. It has affected my self-esteem, my relationships, my career, my thinking, and my insights into people in general.

Please understand: My handicap is not nearly as serious as the disabilities of many others you may have encountered in terms of physical impairment. With help, I overcame a lot of that long before I entered high school. The psychological consequences have been far deeper and have trailed me through the greater part of my life. I have had handicapped friends who envied my ability to get around, climb stairs, walk on rough terrain, and the like.

On the other hand, I have often envied the outward appearance of many of my handicapped friends. None or few of them have such disproportionate legs as I have. Both my legs are shorter than average, making me abnormally short in stature. My right leg has no fat or muscle on it; it is just a skin-covered bone and is two or three inches shorter than the left. It has virtually no muscle power for walking or standing unaided. The difference in length requires me to wear a clumsy shoe, built up with a cork insert and attached to a heavy steel brace that keeps the knee from buckling. The combination has given me an odd walk, which generated acute self-consciousness for most of my early life.

The severity of my disability is largely in my attitude about the body image I project. At times I have been able to forget this. At times it has tortured me. For years and years I have looked for a meaning in this condition.

Perforce, this book will touch on most of the important aspects of my life, but the thread holding it all together will always be my own inquiry as to how my handicap has affected me and the people who relate to me in one way or another, and how it has led me into a more spiritual life.

As a youngster, I spent many long, agonizing hours trying to accept the idea that this was my lot in life. At times I even considered taking the advice of Job's wife, who exhorted her husband to "curse God, and die."

With maturity, however, I began to see how much this handicap has done for me. It was an uphill task, and it could have been made a lot easier for me if relatives, friends, and strangers understood the feelings that a lifelong disability can generate.

There is scarcely a family that does not have at least one member who must cope with the kind of problems I have learned to deal with through years of trial and error—and often with the help of some wonderful people who shared their wisdom with me.

There is scarcely an individual who has not at one time or another had a temporary experience of the feelings I have coped with all through my life.

With this book I hope to share my own learning with other handicapped people of all stripes, with their families, with their friends, their employers, their doctors and therapists, and with the strangers they meet in the course of their daily life. I would like them all to know what a great asset my handicap has been in shaping my character and my relationships.

But I have another purpose. So many people—good people, intelligent people—seem to feel that a physical handicap like mine, which affects only my walking, somehow makes me hard of hearing, half blind, and deficient in intelligence. I think I speak for a large segment of the handicapped when I ask to be treated as an intelligent adult.

These purposes have shaped the format of this book. At the end of each chapter I have appended a section of suggestions to the people who must relate in one way or another to an individual with a disability. I have also included some hard-won observations for the benefit of the handicapped themselves, in the hope that I may spare them a lot of the mental pain I have gone through. I hope it will not seem arrogant that I speak not only as a handicapped person myself, but as a psychotherapist with many years of training and practice behind me.

In order to avoid the clumsy use of "he/she" or "his or her" and the like, I have stayed with the pronoun "he" to represent both genders when appropriate. I have always stood up for the equality and dignity of women—long before the feminist movement—and I beg my feminine readers to understand: Since I myself am a "he," I ask your indulgence in my choice of pronouns.

The incidents in this book are recounted largely from memory, which cannot be perfect. Time sequences and dates may sometimes be inexact. Some names and other identifying details have been changed to protect the people who have played a part in my life. Word-for-word conversations may not have been precisely as given here, but I am quite sure of the content and the meanings behind the words—as I perceived them.

I believe that what is most important is the interplay of feelings between myself and the many, many people I have been fortunate enough to encounter. And I hope, good reader, that your own encounter with this book will be rewarded with an access of insight.

ACKNOWLEDGMENTS

First of all, I want to thank Gwen, my wife, for her tireless support and her constant readiness to help me unravel a multitude of editorial knots with her wise suggestions. She has worked so hard on this book that she has more than earned her byline up front.

I want to thank Joseph Dunn, the Editor-in-Chief of the A.R.E. Press and a veteran journalist, for giving me line-by-line comments and suggestions, which have gone far to improve the quality of my work.

Thanks also to Dr. Mark Thurston, a colleague in the healing profession and the author of several distinguished books, for lending his talents and encouragement to the early shaping of this book.

It has been an extraordinary pleasure to work with these three people in offering my message to the public.

PROLOGUE

Searching for my very first conscious memory, I see myself as a chubby two-year-old, sitting in a wicker wheelchair. I am near a window, dressed warmly for the open air. My legs are in steel braces, sticking straight out.

I am watching the sunrise, and a feeling of ecstatic understanding surges through me. I am in communication with the universe. While I am too little to find words for what I am experiencing, I am filled with the certainty that there is something great and incredibly beautiful out there.

That realization has never left me. It gave me then, and it gives me now, a feeling of specialness—a feeling that, as I came to know, is the birthright of every human being.

CHAPTER
1

THE STIGMA

One of the most eagerly anticipated events of my childhood was the semiannual visit from Daddy O., a distinguished poet and Jungian analyst. When I was little, he would come to see me once a week, but after my mother remarried he would come only at Christmas and on my birthday. My tenth birthday stands out in my memory.

It was a beautiful spring day, and Daddy O. took me for a walk in Central Park, where we chose a bench in the sun. As always, I felt that it was a privilege to be with this warm, important man. While I was basking in his charm, he told me he had a special birthday present for me—an advance copy of *The Mystic Warrior*, a new book he had written in free verse about his own life.

"You can wait till you're a little older to read it," he said. "You'll understand it better then." But, of course, as soon as I was alone, I leafed through the pages eagerly, looking for

1

any mention of myself. I was rewarded with this passage:

> We had thought that our second son would bring us
>   peace . . .
> He is so good-natured, healthy and beautiful,
> A golden boy . . .
>
> Everybody adores him; he is full of laughter and fat
>   chuckles,
> And hardy as a nail . . .
>
> He just begins to walk, and is funny on his feet . . .
>
> But there is no peace: the air in our house has poison
>   in it;
> Though my wife and I muffle our quarrels and lacer-
>   ate each other in secret,
> The air is heavy with a ruined marriage . . .
>
> And one morning I hear the little lad calling me,
> And I go into his room, and he is trying to stand up,
>   clutching on the rods of his crib . . .
> But he cannot stand, he falls back, and looks at me ap-
>   pealingly . . .
>
> I call my wife: something's gone wrong with his legs . . .
> We wait breathlessly for the doctor . . .
> Surely such things happen, but we cannot even think
>   they will happen to us!
> The doctor comes: he tests: yes, it is so,
> It is infantile paralysis . . .
>
> So there between us the golden fruit of our marriage is
>   blasted,
> And we a little see the symbol, the symbol . . .

I was too young to articulate my feelings about those last

two lines, but they crawled their way into my psyche like a virus. It was as though heavy clouds of shame thickened around me, obliterating my identity as a person. My personal disaster apparently meant nothing to my beloved father except as a symbol of his ruined marriage.

The book was inscribed to me, "With much love from Daddy O."

TO PARENTS AND PARENT SURROGATES: The books on parenting will tell you that a child usually blames himself for any troubles he witnesses between his parents. So please, never, never, whether directly or by implication, make a handicapped child feel that his disability is shameful or that it is responsible for bad things happening to members of his family.

Left to their own resources, most children will manage to adapt to a disability. The truly painful part of being handicapped is often the feeling that it somehow disgraces the child. This feeling can easily—and totally unintentionally—be conveyed to him by the most loving, most caring, most important people in his life. Unfortunately the art of parenting was barely understood in the time of my childhood.

I'm sure that my own father, a man with deep feelings, and a psychotherapist as well, never realized what effect his printed words could have on his son. Nor did he understand, in his intense preoccupation with his own problems, how devastated a child might feel on being branded as a symbol of something bad instead of being accepted as a real, special person who is loved unconditionally.

A handicap is a condition of life, like the house one lives in, like the money one's family has, like one's neighbors, or any other given to be reckoned with. It is a condition that calls for adaptation and countermeasures—a challenge, if you will. Meeting that challenge can strengthen and spiritualize the child's character. Explaining this to a child in ways that he can understand may even help him turn that handicap into an asset.

CHAPTER
2

A CHOICE OF DADDIES

Let me go back to the beginning. Among my earliest memories are the frequent afternoon "naps" I took (never sleeping) on my mother's big bed. We were in our new Manhattan apartment on East 81st Street, where we had moved after my father left us. Lying there, I often wondered why he wasn't living with us any more and why he only came to see us for dinner on Sundays.

During my afternoon naps we were often visited by Dr. Stark, a nice young family doctor who had set up his practice in the front parlor of my maternal grandmother's brownstone house on East 79th Street—the house I so often visited with my mother, my father (before their divorce), and my older brother Ralph.

I remember how the good doctor would lie on the bed with me during his visits and sing songs from his own childhood—old favorites like "Swanee River," or "The Village

Blacksmith," and others—some that I have never heard since then. One of them in particular fascinated me with its bouncy rhythm and the images it evoked in my childish mind. It went like this:

> Get away from the window,
> You saucy little devil!
> Get away from the window that I say!
> Come around tomorrow night
> And there's sure to be a fight.
> Get away from the window today!

One day, when I was around three-and-a-half years old, my young, pretty mother told me that she was going away for a weekend vacation and that our housekeeper would look after me while she was gone. My brother Ralph was away at a boarding school in New Jersey. I didn't at all like the idea of being left without any family, but I swallowed my objections.

I have a very clear image of myself taking my routine nap in my mother's room when she returned from her vacation. That nice Dr. Stark was with her; he was almost like one of the family.

Lying on my mom's big bed, I watched curiously as the doctor began unpacking his suitcase in her bedroom. What did that mean? I wondered. I became even more curious when he drew a pair of military hairbrushes from his luggage and began brushing his hair in front of the mirror above my mom's dresser. Presently he laid the brushes down on the dresser top and turned his head toward me.

"You can call me Daddy now," he said.

"I *have* a Daddy," was my immediate response, but I was strangely troubled by his words.

"Well, now you have two daddies," he said, "Daddy S. and Daddy O. I'm Daddy S."

I could not bring myself to offend this friendly man by telling him that I really didn't want another daddy. But at the same time I felt challenged in my loyalty to my own father. The best response I could come up with was to remain impassively silent, a strategy that clung to me well into my adult life.

A few nights later I had a dream—the earliest dream in my conscious memory bank. I was walking through a woods at twilight and came out at the side of a narrow dirt road. There was a peaceful, pastoral feeling about the scene, quite different from our New York City environment.

Across the road and up on a grassy mound was a trim white house with a soft, friendly light shining out through the windows. As I stood there, breathing in the tranquillity of the setting, the front door of the house opened and a procession of men in business suits came walking out single file. There were at least a hundred of them. They walked down the embankment to the edge of the road, where they lined up, side by side, facing me.

No word was spoken, but I knew exactly what this was all about: I had to choose from those hundred men the one man I wanted to be my daddy.

Daddy O. was in the line-up, and so was Daddy S. Another man I recognized was Arthur Gleason—"Uncle Arthur" to me—a family friend who, with his regally beautiful wife, often exchanged visits with us. Uncle Arthur, a rugged, comfortable-looking man with an outdoorsy air about him, always took time during his visits for a personal chat with me. He was altogether the kind of person I would have been proud to have as my daddy. All things being equal, I'm quite sure I would have chosen him.

But all things were not equal. There was my father, and there was my stepfather, both of them looking at me with patient expectancy.

There was only one way to resolve this paralyzing love-

and-loyalty conflict: I woke up.

Daddy O.'s Sunday visits persisted for a month or two after my mother remarried, and I remember the twisty feelings I would have sitting at the dinner table between my two fathers. Perhaps some of the grown-ups felt funny, too, for Daddy O.'s visits soon tapered off to a semiannual frequency. It was somewhere around this time that the Night Visitors first made their appearance.

───────

TO PARENTS AND SURROGATES: Please be especially careful to spare the handicapped child a conflict of family loyalties. While this advice holds good for any small child, the one with negative feelings about himself is especially vulnerable.

One of the great fears of any child with a conspicuous disability is the fear of abandonment. In many early cultures such children were taken to the woods or the desert and left to die; the males would be useless as hunters and warriors, while the females would never be desirable mates or proficient housekeepers. Worse yet, in some cultures a flawed child was a badge of disgrace. So the fears of little children in those cultures had a very real basis. That same fear in a modified form may well be a kind of atavistic phenomenon.

In today's somewhat more civilized culture, a child is not so much afraid of being abandoned in the woods or left to die in the desert as he is terrified of being thrown on his own resources when loved adults leave him—especially if his resources are depleted by a handicap. The child who already may think of himself as flawed in his body is likely to feel unworthy of love and caring from the adults he depends on. Pressures to undermine his loyalty to a parent or surrogate diminish his already low self-esteem and may give him a very shaky start in life.

CHAPTER
3

THE NIGHT VISITORS

I was not yet four when the Little Old Man started coming into my bedroom. He never came when I was lying on my side—only when I was on my back. But that was pretty usual.

He was a very small old man, and he was a sort of luminous white. His face, his long, pointy beard, his hands, and his clothing were all that same whitish color—even his cap, which had the shape of a dunce cap.

He seemed gentle and friendly enough. Just as I was nearing the verge of sleep, he would pad in soundlessly, as if he didn't want to startle me. After positioning himself at the head of my bed, he would lean down, grasp my temples between his delicate hands and gently turn me over on my side. I have never to this day quite understood why he didn't like me to sleep on my back. Was there, perhaps, something that he didn't want me to see?

I was not really afraid of him, but neither was I quite comfortable with this ritual. Why didn't I tell my parents about his visits? Even at that young age, I think I anticipated that they would dismiss my story as imagination or dream stuff. But I knew that the Little Old Man was real. I could see him clearly and I could feel his hands on my head, coaxing my whole body to turn over.

I soon realized that if I learned to fall asleep on my side, my visitor would not come into the room. With secret effort, I acquired the habit of turning over by myself as soon as I began to feel sleepy. My little old friend's visits were then confined to those rare nights when I forgot to turn over. I finally trained myself to the point where his appearances were terminated altogether. But then I had another kind of visitation.

One night after turning over on my side, facing the wall, I was shocked into wakefulness by the sight of three demonic faces. They had long, long necks (about two feet long, in retrospect) that protruded from the wall in an upward curve. Each head was topped by a pair of small horns and further disfigured with hideous excrescences. Each head was a different phosphorescent color—one red, one blue, one green; and in spite of their similarities, each face had its own fiendish individuality.

They didn't look at me. Their motionless stare was fixed straight ahead, but I knew that their purpose was to terrorize me. And once more I refrained from calling out to my parents. Instead, I simply stared back at my Night Visitors in fear and fascination until they faded and dissolved into the dark air.

I don't know how long these secret staring matches continued, but one night I experimented by turning onto my left side, away from the wall beside my bed. This took some doing, as I was by now accustomed to sleeping on my right. But that night the visitors left me alone. If they were there, I never saw them. Nor was I bothered by any sense of their presence.

It did not take me very long to learn to go to sleep with my back to the wall, and for a good while I was left in peace. But then a baby brother, Louis, was born, and presently I was shifted to another bedroom. My bed was now positioned so that when I slept on my left side, as I had trained myself to do, I would be facing the wall. But by this time I was retiring at night without giving any thought to my frightening visitors. On my first night in my new room, however, just as I was beginning to get sleepy, there they were.

This shifting back and forth from right side to left side and back went on for a few years. Every time my older brother Ralph came home from boarding school, the bed arrangements were likely to be changed. And every time I slipped up, the faces came back to remind me that there was still malevolence in my inner world. But by the time I was nine years old, I had trained myself so well that I was able to put them out of my life.

I enjoyed about two years of nights without apparitions. Then, when I was eleven, my family took me to the Poconos for the summer. By this time I had pretty much forgotten about the hideous faces. So on the first night there, I went to bed in my accustomed way, turning onto my left side before going to sleep.

There was a blank white wall facing me, and after a while a new kind of vision materialized between the wall and my bed—an indescribably beautiful Goddess with a divine luminosity emanating from every part of her. I was filled with a deep sense of peace and gratitude—gratitude because I knew that she was an immortal and that from here on I would be under her protection.

All this was many, many years ago, and I have gone through life wondering about the meaning of those Night Visitors. As a psychotherapist, I have tried to look on them as fantasies reflecting the complex of distressing situations that developed in my early years, but no interpretation has ever emerged that isn't forced.

I finally got a strong feeling that I should stop analyzing and simply accept that culminating vision as a beautiful gift, with all the inner euphoria it has brought me. The image of this Goddess has stayed with me through the years. Whenever I send up a prayer, that childhood vision comes into my spirit in all its pristine serenity.

TO PARENTS AND PARENT SURROGATES: I know that many, many children go through experiences fully as troubling or as scary as the ones I remember. I know, too, that they rarely mention these experiences to their parents—or even to their brothers and sisters. These children are in need of help, and the grown-ups in their lives would do well to learn when to volunteer that help without being asked.

How do you know when to offer your help? There are certain signs that should put you on the alert. Does your child resist going to bed at night? Does he avoid certain places in the home or outside? Does he seem preoccupied at mealtimes or when you try to talk to him? Does he have nightmares? Is he doing poorly at school? Any of these signs are worth investigating; a cluster of them warrants your all-out concern.

These signs may signal any of a number of problems— fear of abandonment, for example, or fear of being caught in some forbidden activity, or fear of abuse by some member of the family. They may also be the first clues that your child is being visited by frightening entities. Whatever these symptoms may be, they are calls for help.

What can you do about it? First of all, try to get your child to talk—not in a formal, let's-sit-down-and-talk-this-over sort of way, which in itself can be frightening, but in as casual a manner as you can manage. For example, while playing a game you might bring up the subject of childhood worries. Talk about some of your own worries and fears when you were little and those that you know other children have—worries about bad dreams, fears that their parents might leave them, fears of punishment for doing something they know they shouldn't have done, anxieties about spirits coming to visit them—whether they are spirits that like to help children or spirits that want to scare them.

Encourage your child to talk about any experiences he might have had with problems like these, and gradually draw him out. If he mentions demons or other frightening apparitions, listen sympathetically. Reassure him that he is safe under your protection. Tell him emphatically that if he is ever frightened by spirits, the best thing he can do for himself is to ask you to help him. Above all, never, *never* dismiss his accounts as dreams or imagination. Instead of reassuring him, that approach will only make him feel that you don't understand.

If he persistently resists your approaches, it would be a good idea to get professional help. At his early stage of life, a capable, caring therapist—one who doesn't scoff—might save him from years of anxiety and fear.

Yes, professional help is expensive. But let your child's need persuade you to examine your priorities.

CHAPTER
4

BONDING WITH DADDY S.

Daddy S. had hardly taken his place in our family when he firmly and determinedly took charge of me as my doctor. I had acquired polio at the age of fourteen months, and the standard treatment in those days was to immobilize the affected limbs. As a result, I spent more than six months of my babyhood lying in an enormous plaster cast. This, of course, allowed my leg muscles to deteriorate. When I was able to walk, it was only with two leg braces and a pair of crutches.

Daddy S., a family physician and surgeon, had thought my problem through and developed some ideas about the potentials of the human body that were a bit ahead of his time. He kept my braces off during the day, encouraging me to get around any way I could, including crawling. This not only freed my legs from restriction but gave them a chance to exercise.

He put the braces back on me at night, however, to correct the deviations in the alignment of my limbs. Under his care I gradually improved. As I continued to grow, Daddy S. encouraged me to discard the brace on my left leg, which still had some muscle and was growing faster than the right. With further encouragement, I discarded one of my crutches and finally exchanged the other one for a cane.

Daddy S. even performed a few minor operations on me at home, with my mother acting as his assistant. I have a vague memory of struggling to push away a white mask he was holding over my nose, making me feel that I couldn't breathe. But a moment later I was watching a procession of rafts floating down the Hudson River in single file. In the center of each raft was a white rabbit, sitting quietly on its haunches. Then I woke up and it was all over. Even today I often use the image of the white rabbits drifting down the river to hypnotize myself.

Daddy S. wanted the best for me. He took me to some of the top orthopedic specialists in New York to tap their expertise. I still have a dim memory that must go back to age four or five, a memory of lying on an examining table under bright lights with a ring of venerable doctors around me. They were pumping my limbs up and down and giving their opinions to Daddy S. He listened, nodding politely, but his face was furrowed into a frown. I found myself developing a deep liking for this man who had all but displaced my original father.

When mainstream medicine floundered on my case, Daddy S. was not above trying alternative methods that most doctors considered outlandish in those days. And I'm sure some of them were!

I remember being taken to a Scottish healer who assured Daddy S., "I'll have that boy on roller-skates in three months." His treatment consisted of applying drops of a brownish liquid to my spine while he sang:

Oh, it's neece to get up in the mornin'
   When the sun begins to sheen
At four or five or six o'clock
   In the good ol' summer teem.

But when the clouds are ragin'
   And it's murky over your 'ead,
Oh, it's neece to get up in the mornin'
   But it's neecer to stay in bed.

"Neecer" we should have stayed away from that friendly quack!

Though I was too young to articulate my feelings, I was impressed by my stepfather's unremitting efforts on my behalf. But I was also distressed by the way he ignored my feelings in certain situations. Whenever he took me to the office of a doctor or a therapist, for example, he would insist on taking off my shoes and braces, and even stripping me down to my underwear in the waiting room—so that we wouldn't waste any of his colleague's time when we were called in. At such times I almost hated him.

It was nearly as bad when we were riding together by bus. Long before we reached our destination he would make me lock my braces, disregarding the fact that I could do this in an instant, or that he was inviting public attention to my stiffened limbs.

Sometimes Daddy S. could get so boorish that our whole family felt he was making a public spectacle of us. Whenever we went to a Chinese restaurant, for example, he would ask the waiter, "We get licee with dinner?"

"Certainly, sir," was the typical reply. "It's included in the dinner."

"O.K. You bling licee with soupee."

"Yes, sir."

At such moments, the rest of us would look at each other in acute mortification. My mother and brothers seemed to get over it quickly, but the bad feeling would cling to me for a long time.

Daddy S. lost points with me, all right; but in retrospect I would still rate him as an outstanding parent.

Daddy O., meanwhile, had moved to Glendale, California, and my brother Ralph soon went to live with him there. I began to receive long, beautiful letters from both of them, supporting me in my ambition to write poems and stories, like Daddy O., and offering me instructive criticism of my clumsy efforts.

In Daddy O.'s letters there were vivid descriptions of the great climate, the lovely people, the spectacular scenery. He wrote eloquently about the development of a portable typewriter with a standard keyboard, and about a new taste treat called Eskimo Pie, a block of ice cream wrapped in chocolate.

Quite casually he would mention "Mother O." I gathered that he was remarried to this artist, who signed her paintings Gertrude S. Gertrude. This was the first I knew that I now had two mothers as well as two fathers. But little did I know at this juncture that Mother O. was later to generate new excitements in my life, as well as new conflicts—not with my biological mother, but with my Daddy O. She began sending me charming letters that were written in a bold, very large kind of calligraphy. I fell in love with her long before I ever met her.

In New York we were also making some important moves. Daddy S. rented a spacious office on West 86th Street, and not long after that we all moved into a six-room apartment on 83rd Street, just a few city blocks from the office and a few steps from Riverside Park.

We called one room the "playroom." Daddy S. furnished it with a big workbench, a couple of stools, a vise, an abundance of carpentry tools and a lot of ideas. Over the years, as children, we spent many happy hours making things and experimenting with our chemistry set.

One day, as I was passing the playroom, I noticed that the door was closed and an unusually bright light was shining through the cracks. I called in to my younger brother Louis, who was the only person who could be in that room. There was no answer.

"Let me in!" I shouted several times, but still there was no answer. My mother heard me and rushed to my side. "Open the door!" she commanded. A frightened little boy opened up. A small chemical fire was blazing on the workbench. Mom and I were able to put it out quickly, but not before it had left some scars on the table.

I thought of the terrible things that could have happened but didn't, and a familiar sense of warmth came over me. I got this feeling in many other situations throughout my life: Someone or something was watching over us.

For my benefit, Daddy S. installed a diathermy machine in his office to treat me with high-frequency electromagnetic radiation. The school bus would let me off at his office every weekday afternoon for a half-hour treatment, after which he or his nurse would walk me home. I preferred going with him, because we would always stop at Wasself's drugstore for an ice-cream soda.

Secondarily, I was proud to be in his company. He was a stocky man with a springy step that exuded energy and authority. I made many grown-up friends on these walks and in his waiting room, including a nice lady who regularly invited me to her apartment, where she regaled me with refreshments and caramels and lots of praise.

That was the period before hi-tech had got into orthopedics and orthotics. On our walks I often saw persons with one extremely foreshortened leg walking on a metal rocker that was attached to the shoe on the affected limb by a vertical iron bar. The sight of it freaked me out. I made a powerful resolution to avoid this fate by keeping my growth down so that there wouldn't be such a difference between my right leg and my left. I told myself that I would rather be a shorty than walk on such a cloppering contraption.

My resolution worked. At least I think it did. I grew up to a height of five feet and four inches. At this height, my right leg is only a couple of inches shorter than my left, and I can wear custom-made shoes to compensate. I still like to believe that this was my own victory of mind over matter.

Daddy S. often took me along when he made his morning rounds at two or three hospitals and at apartments where he had housebound patients. We would be picked up in a taxi driven by Mr. Griffin, a genial, talkative Irishman who would regale me with stories and homespun philosophy while Daddy S. was looking after his patients.

This energetic Daddy would often take me, alone or with my brothers, down to the waterfront below Riverside Park, where we would build a fire and roast potatoes on sticks—mickeys, we called them.

Up in the park he would negotiate with other children to get me into their games. If they were playing softball, for instance, he would arrange for me to bat the ball while a teammate would do the running for me. He also took me to the circus, to children's shows, to the Museum of Natural History, and to "real" baseball games at the Yankee Stadium.

I remember watching the mighty Babe Ruth once and waiting for him to do something spectacular. Daddy S. explained to me that when the bases were loaded, the visiting team was deliberately pitching foul balls to him. This forced the Babe to walk to first base when he might have hit a home run. The maneuver, called "walking," made me very angry, not only at the visiting team but at the system, which condoned such unfairness. The Babe finally had his chance, however, and I was sadly disappointed when he hit only a three-bagger.

My mother also liked to take me to the park, and my activities then would be quite different. We would sit on a bench while she would read to me, or she would crochet while I plied her with questions. By the time I was seven or eight I would often wander off by myself. On my own I rarely tried to make friends with other children. My ingrained fear of rejection made me cautious.

Instead, I would gravitate toward a particular bench where I knew I would find four special friends, aged seventy-five to ninety, who gathered there every nice day to trade memories and opinions. The senior member of this group was Mr. Yeager, a very compact old man with a neat gray beard and a derby hat. He could tell great stories about the Civil War.

But my very special friend was Mr. Appleby, who, to my astonishment, could spit brown. One Christmas he gave me an erector set, a set of metal parts that fit together so you could construct things with them. Mr. Appleby smoked a pipe and chewed tobacco, but I never connected that with the brown saliva.

I think these four old men gave me a sense of belonging, an identity as a member of their impressive group. I remember them with affection. More than that, I could enjoy their company without any sense of competition.

———————

TO PARENTS AND SURROGATES: I know that many children would have no qualms about exposing their bodies to strangers; but a handicapped child who is struggling with a depressing body image can be acutely distressed at being forced to make a public exhibition of his infirmities. Any adult in charge of a disabled child should be sure to learn the child's feelings and respect his special sensitivity.

Both daddies were trying, each in his own way, to be good to me, but the result was to polarize my feelings. And it surely was no help when grown-ups would ask me, "Which daddy do you like better?" It was a question I tried my best not to answer, because each daddy was giving me something special, something that defied comparison.

Daddy S. was the one who was always there for me—with medical help, with financial support, with material gifts, with family feeling. He was the one who understood my disability on the medical level and helped me find ways of overcoming it.

Daddy O. was there for me in another way. Though I saw him infrequently, he was the one who encouraged me to dream, to create, to become intimate with the great poets and dreamers of the past, to delve into psychological and metaphysical territories. How could I compare them? Pressure to choose which daddy I preferred could only make me feel disloyal to one or the other.

———

TO DOCTORS, HEALERS, AND OTHERS: Such remarks as "I'll have that child on roller-skates in three months" are a sure way to build the handicapped child's hopes up to a cruel letdown. In the same category is the advice the superintendent of our Manhattan apartment house gave me: "If anybody says you're handicapped, you just give 'em a good, swift kick in the pants!" And the exhortations of a well-meaning uncle of mine, who assured me, when I was eleven years old, "Don't let a little handicap hold you back. You can be anything you want to be!"

Remarks like that and those of the Scottish healer and the apartment superintendent are made, certainly, in a spirit of helpfulness, but they usually have just the opposite effect. Why try to convince the handicapped child that he can do things far beyond what's possible for him? Why not, instead, tell him about the wonderful things he really *can* do? Maybe he can become a great swimmer or a canoeist or a musician or a famous doctor. There is a virtually limitless menu to choose from. So help him build a positive image of himself.

CHAPTER 5

WHAT ABOUT GOD?

Daddy S. rarely spoke to me about God, and neither, as far as I can remember, did my mother. When I was around seven or eight, however, I read a children's version of both the Old and the New Testaments. While I was browsing in this book one night and Daddy S. was relaxing in a nearby armchair, I asked him, "Do you believe in God?"

I was shocked when he replied, gently but honestly, that he didn't believe in God or Heaven or Hell. When the shock wore off, I found myself feeling sorry for him. I wished that I could help him, because I was sure that God existed and that Hell was real. I had seen those demonic faces on my bedroom wall, and I knew that they could only have come from Hell. I had also ingested the teachings of Jesus and was convinced that this wonderful man was speaking truth.

What puzzled me was that Daddy S., though he described himself as a nonbeliever, nevertheless loved to observe some of the Jewish religious rituals in his own way. Every Friday night, the beginning of the Jewish Sabbath, we would light the two candles on the mantelpiece in the dining room, and we would have fish for dinner. We celebrated, in an informal way, both Chanukah and Christmas, which was very nice for us kids because we got presents on both occasions. Furthermore, Daddy S. put me into Sunday school, but hardly ever went to synagogue himself.

One day, however, while Daddy S. and I were walking home from his office, he told me that we were going to stop at a synagogue to hear a service. On the way he explained that this day was Yom Kippur, the Jewish Day of Atonement.

Sitting next to him during the service, I was awestruck by the atmosphere of solemnity pervading this house of God. After a while I turned to look at my stepfather. I was astonished, and a little fearful, at the sight of large tears rolling down his cheeks.

I had never seen him weep, and I knew that he had told me he was not a religious man. Yet here was evidence that I could only feel—evidence of a genuine spirituality in this nonbeliever. Was he somehow tapping into a deep well of divinity? I could not put my perception into words, but it brought up my own experience of connection with an indescribable creative energy that stays with me as my first memory.

Daddy S. came from a devout Jewish family, though you never would have guessed it from his modern clothes, his gusty speech or his manner. On one occasion he took my mother and me to a gathering at the home of *his* mother, who lived in a walk-up on the Lower East Side.

I couldn't help wondering how this tiny, tired-looking woman could have given birth to twelve strapping adults— not just my Daddy S., but eleven others who called themselves my aunts and uncles. I was deeply moved by their love and devotion to their Mama, as well as to each other. I record the occasion here because somehow I knew that this happy gathering, like the tears on my stepfather's cheeks, was a religious experience.

But I must confess, rather sheepishly, that what stands out most clearly in my conscious memory of that day is what I saw from the window: a horse-drawn streetcar! Even at my very tender age I was curiously impressed by this relic of another era. I had seen streetcars with overhead trolleys and streetcars that drew their power through a slot in the pavement, but now I suddenly knew the meaning of the word "horsepower."

I don't usually like to talk about this incredible sight today because I fear it will make me look as old as Methuselah. And maybe I am. Sometimes I wonder if that streetcar was a flashback memory of a previous lifetime.

The apparent conflict between my stepfather's words and his religious behavior not only puzzled me, but it started me thinking about my discovery that there are many faiths in the world. Daddy O., on my seventh birthday, had presented me with a book called *The Children's Homer*. It was written by Padraic Colum, an Irish poet who was one of Daddy O.'s good friends, and it was compellingly illustrated by Willy Pogany.

This enchanting tale of the Trojan War and the wanderings of Odysseus is still one of my most treasured books. As a seven-year-old child, I read it over and over, and then collected everything I could find on the Greek gods and goddesses.

Some of these books, like Bulfinch's *Mythology*, also contained stories from other religions, especially the tales of Valhalla, the home of those exciting Scandinavian deities.

Which is the true faith? I wondered. Should I be praying to Jehovah or Jesus or Zeus or Wotan or Buddha or Allah? And if I prayed to the wrong one, would the true God be angry with me? When I tried to discuss my puzzlement with people who claimed to know, I got very positive answers about which religion was true. But the answers didn't agree with each other. I prayed to a nameless God for an answer that would make sense to me.

When I reached the age of eleven, the appearance of the beautiful Goddess at my bedside finally gave me my own answer. As usual, it was not an answer that I could put into words, but it planted some kind of conviction in me that started to dissolve my confusion without my knowing why. Even today I feel like a very spiritual person. But when I am asked, as in a hospital admissions office, what my religion is, I reply, "That's between me and my Creator. Just leave it blank."

Seeing those tears roll down my stepfather's cheeks in synagogue was a powerful experience for me. Though I did not know why he was grieving, I could sense the depth of his feeling. Neither of us ever talked about it, but the bond between the macho doctor and the baffled little boy was sealed—sealed with a spiritual love.

When my thirteenth birthday approached, I revolted at my stepfather's plan to have me go through the bar mitzvah ceremony, the Jewish equivalent of confirmation. I held out stubbornly for months, but as the date approached, my stepfather's relatives began putting the pressure on me. They would take me aside, one by one, and gently tell me that I really ought to do this for Daddy S., who had done so much for me. "Do it for him," they kept urging me. And I finally gave in.

The rabbi, who by now was a frequent guest at our dinner table, said he was pleased, but that at this late date there really was no time for me to learn the meaning of the ceremonial words. He said the best I could do would be to memorize the sounds of the Hebrew words, including the cues he would give me in Hebrew, and recite my part in a clear voice.

A year or two before that time I had written a book of poems titled *Lyrics to the Olympian Deities,* which I peddled energetically to all my friends and members of my families. In the course of my research, I had compiled a list of the Greek gods and goddesses, which I kept in my trousers pocket because I was constantly enlarging it.

At the service, I looked around and was cowed by the number of familiar faces in the congregation. I prayed to my special Goddess to keep me from stumbling. And while I was praying I heard the rabbi intoning the sounds, "Yah a mode bar mitzvah"—my cue.

Still praying, I got to my feet and limped to the rabbi's side at the podium. As soon as we started, I slipped a hand into my trousers pocket and clutched my list of gods and goddesses, pleading with my special Goddess to make this occasion a success.

It was a responsive ceremony, and I soon realized that my prayer was taking effect; I came in on every cue with just the right Hebrew words, having no idea what either of us were talking about.

A few minutes later, as we were all leaving the synagogue, my relatives gathered around me on the sidewalk to hug and kiss and congratulate me. Several of them said they had never heard the bar mitzvah ceremony rendered "*with so much expression!!!*" (Italics and exclamation points are mine.)

———————

TO PARENTS, SURROGATES, AND RELATIVES: What does a grown-up do when a child asks about religion? Be aware that he is asking for answers that may stay with him for life. When the question comes from a handicapped child, you can be pretty certain that he has a special reason to want some answers. Why isn't his body whole and sound, like everybody else's? Did he do something bad that made God angry? And anyway, does God really exist? If He does, why is there so much disagreement about Him?

These are tough questions indeed, and they call for good answers. There certainly is no one answer for everybody, but you can give your child the answers you feel comfortable with. Let me suggest a few that may possibly fit in with your ideas.

In the first place, you can tell your child your own feelings about God, even if you don't believe there is a God. I think my stepfather was right in telling me how he felt, but he could have gone a lot further. He could have said that people have worshiped God in one way or another since long before civilization. They have given different names to Him and pictured Him the way they like to think He is.

The Jewish God, as depicted in the Bible, is a stern but loving father, while the Christian God is gentle and forgiving. I'm convinced that it doesn't matter whether you think of Him as Zeus or Krishna or Odin, or as Gaia or Mother Earth. What matters is whether you believe in some creative force or energy that helps to explain why we're all here.

One of the most comforting answers a parent can give a child is that people don't die—they just leave their tired bodies and go someplace where they prepare to come back to earth as babies. If you can sincerely tell a handicapped child that there may be some divine reason for his disability, you can also give him the hope for a more perfect body the next time around.

But if you, yourself, are agnostic, I would suggest that you ask yourself whether telling your child you don't believe in God—and leaving it at that—may be a way of depriving him of some deep and joyful experiences. A better approach, I think, might be to tell him that people have always believed in some creator that put us here for a reason. Then ask him what *he* thinks about God. You may instill in him a wonderment at the miracle of life and how it took millions of years to perfect a body like his own—and to enable that body to think and feel and act.

If your child then, using his imagination, offers some explanations of his own or even a story of creation, encourage him to think about it often. You may even tell him about some of the beliefs of other people throughout history and around the world. Finally, you might assure him that he will find the answer within himself.

CHAPTER
6

"RUN WITH ME TO THE TREE"

When the preschool years rolled in, my parents placed me in a little private nursery a few blocks from my home. It was here that I encountered the first signs of prejudice because I was lame. At least that was the only reason I could figure out.

Most of the children seemed to accept me as one of them despite my disability. The teachers, however, were constantly finding fault with me and excluding me from activities I could master as well as any other kid. I understood why I could not join in games that involved running, jumping, or dancing, but I didn't understand why I was not allowed to sit with the others in a circle to tell stories or play word games.

On another front, I remember getting into a heated argument with a schoolmate. He threatened to have his father beat me up and dwelt on what a frightening giant his father was. But I was not put down.

"My father could lick your father easy," I said contemptuously.

"Yeah? Well, my father is as high as you and me put together!"

"Oh yeah? Well, my father is so high that if he stood up, his head would hit the ceiling and there would be blood all over!"

My classmate refused to be outdone. "If *my* father stood up, his head would go right through the ceiling and everything would fall down!"

How could I top that one? I thought a moment, then drew myself up to my full height and delivered the coup de grâce. "I," I said, "have *two* fathers!" I could see by the look on his face that my adversary was crushed. I watched him as he turned away and walled off. It was the first time I felt that there was a payoff in having two fathers.

A few days later, I got into serious trouble for wiping my nose on my shirtsleeve, as I had seen several of the other kids do (because Kleenex® had not yet come on the market and my handkerchief was used up). The teacher in charge grabbed my arm, told me that I was disgusting, and ordered me to go home for a clean handkerchief.

I left the school scared and crying—scared because I was still walking with two crutches and a brace, and crying because I was finally convinced that the teachers didn't like me. As I walked on, I was thinking about this and all the other incidents in which I had felt singled out. This led me to an unfortunate generalization: Teachers just don't like lame kids.

It was my first venture onto the city streets by myself, and there were two or three crossings to contend with. Fortunately, I met my mother on the way. She marched me right back to the school, where she charged into the classroom and laid my teacher out with all the fury of a lioness defending her cub.

I remember hoping for some assurance from my mother that I was not a bad boy, but I think I understood: She was probably too wrapped up in her anger at the teacher for putting my life in danger. What I needed from her would have called for a change of mood. Her moods usually translated instantly into verbal or body language, and her emphatic movements as we walked home hand in hand left me wondering whether I was just as bad as that teacher.

The next thing I knew, I was in a Montessori school, where children were encouraged to educate themselves with minimal adult guidance. I recall a very important event in the classroom there. My teacher was showing me pictures in a book. One of the pictures showed a little boy and a little girl running hand in hand toward a tree. The picture tapped into a wistfulness within me that always surfaced when I was reminded that I could not run and jump like other children.

I was not really listening to what my teacher was telling me, but I finally realized that she was calling my attention to the printed words accompanying the picture. I looked at them, and a light went on inside of me as I suddenly understood what they said:

> Run with me
> To the tree.

I spoke the words aloud, bringing a nod and a smile to the face of my teacher. I confined my exhilaration to a shout: "I can read!" And I was launched on one of the greatest activities of my life—reading. There are a lot of answers in the books.

TO TEACHERS: I hardly need to say anything here against prejudice and discrimination; by now all parents and people who work with children are familiar with the message disseminated by the media on this subject. I do have an approach to offer to loving and concerned teachers when they are confronted with a situation in which all the children except the handicapped one can participate. For example:

Tell the exceptional child that you want to give him a special and important job. If the children are involved in a competition, let him be the referee. If it is a dance to a recorded piece, put him in charge of the music.

With love and ingenuity you can always find some way to make the handicapped child a significant contributor. This not only helps him feel better about his disability, but also gives the other kids a hands-on experience of accepting the handicapped into their society.

TO PARENTS AND SURROGATES: Anger is always a destructive emotion, but there are times when it is called for—such as when a grown-up expresses her prejudices by needlessly endangering the life of a child. My mother was an expert at venting her anger, but she was also an expert at demonstrating love. I think her outburst at the teacher was unquestionably justified. Her more important job, however, was to heal the psychological wound that had been inflicted on me. I had to wait for that treatment until her anger spent itself.

The child who is coping with shame about his body image is always looking for assurances from others that he is liked and valued. The best kind of help you can give him when he is a victim of prejudice is to hold a loving conversation with him. Explain to him that some people say and do mean things because they don't know any better; maybe they've been treated badly themselves when they were kids, and they're full of hate. Explain that while you and he can't change other people, you can help him change himself so that he won't let other people's prejudices get him down.

Make it clear to your child that you are on his side and that you know what a good person he is. Tell him that you will always be there to protect him. Try to convince him that most people are good and that he will always have friends who love him.

A nice follow-up to such a chat would be to invite a bunch of friendly kids to join him in a party or a pleasant outing, with Mom and/or Dad present to show him what you mean.

You may think of many other ways to make your point. This is the kind of situation you can turn to good account by using it to fight prejudice and strengthen the bonds of love.

CHAPTER
7

ME AND MISS LEE

When I reached second grade I was placed in P.S. 9, a neighborhood public school. I got along fine with my teacher and my classmates, and I was very pleased to be treated the same as all the other boys. But not for long.

At my overprotective mother's behest, I feel sure, the teacher appointed a friendly classmate to accompany me whenever I had to leave the room—even if it was only to go to the bathroom. The idea, I imagine, was to make sure I didn't have a fall. I couldn't see how Stuart could have prevented me from hurting myself, but I liked him a lot. I liked his face, his manner, and the way his ears stuck way out. Only I didn't like being monitored.

Very early in the term the alarm sounded for a fire drill, and Stuart dutifully stayed at my side to "protect" me as we went down a flight of stairs and out into the street. In spite of my reservations about being supervised, I enjoyed the

excitement of the drill, and Stuart and I entertained ourselves by pretending it was a real conflagration.

After I told my mother about the fire drill, she had a
serious talk with my teacher, and I could only guess what it
meant. Next time the alarm sounded I was instructed to remain in the classroom while all the other children—
including Stuart—rushed to "safety" in the street.

I sat at my desk listening to the commotion outside and
wondering what would happen if this was a real fire. While
everybody else would be allowed to run to safety, I would be
trapped in the classroom, doomed to be burned alive. Hu-
miliating!

My mother always picked me up for lunch, and one day I
unwittingly gave her a bad shock. As I started down the
stairs, I lost my footing. I began tumbling, head over heels,
as it seemed, and was acutely aware of my mother scream-
ing, "Stop! Stop!" as she chased after me.

I remember being more amused than afraid, and thinking how ridiculous it was to tell me to stop when that was
totally impossible. When I finally did come to a stop, I found
myself sitting on the lowermost step, laughing uncontrolla-
bly. That was my last day in P.S. 9.

Overruling my protests, my protective mother placed me
in a school that had a special class "for crippled children,"
as it was then designated. The setting was a classroom in
P.S. 54, situated on the ground floor in a corner of the school
nearest the entrance. It was accessed by four or five steps.

All the grades were assembled into this one room, so that
it was like an old-fashioned, one-room country school
within a large city school. Each child had almost all the same
classmates until he graduated, and we had the same teacher
through the years.

In my first term there I was actually picked up by a horse-
drawn coach with two lengthwise benches inside. It was
manned by a strict lady who had some difficulty keeping

her charges from laughing and moving about. As the coach made stop after stop to pick up the children, I was impressed by the range of disabilities my classmates presented.

Finally the coach stopped at 104th Street and Amsterdam Avenue to discharge some eighteen children of varying ages and impairments. It was painful for me to watch them limping and hobbling and pulling themselves up the stairs by grasping the handrails to get into the building. One girl had to be carried up in a wheelchair.

I lagged behind as long as I was allowed to because I did not want to be identified as a member of this ungainly troupe, as I then perceived them. I was still using two braces and two crutches at this time, and I was acutely self-conscious.

Across the street from the school was a dreary red building with some lettering chiseled into it over the entrance. The letters spelled out, "A Home for the Aged and Indigent Females of the City of New York." Somehow the combination of "Crippled Children" and "Aged and Indigent Females" worked on my insides, turning everything into a somber gray.

I have memories of a very good-looking woman who visited the classroom frequently, and of the great feeling of pride that welled up in me whenever she came through the door. This beautiful woman was my mother.

It didn't take me long to become comfortable—there were so many really great kids who could talk my language. I soon had several good friends. And one enemy.

William was a bully. He was a good deal bigger than I, and far less handicapped. It was not long before he singled me out as his punching bag. Every morning as we were settling into our room, William would come over to me and start punching me, right in sight of the whole class. Several of the girls told him to pick on someone his size, but nothing stopped him.

It got so that I went to school each morning with a growing anticipation of a pummeling. Finally, at dinner one evening, I told my parents about William. Daddy S.'s answer was simple: "Give him back two for one." I protested that he was twice my size and much stronger, but Daddy S. just repeated, "Two for one. Two for one."

My stepfather's exhortations only increased my feeling of helplessness, and I went to school next day with a growing anxiety. William was there, and he came toward me with the same bullying look in his eyes.

I felt a blazing rage surge up inside of me, and suddenly I lunged at William, pummeling him with both hands, using all my strength. I saw the astonished look on his face, but it quickly turned to a look of fear. And from that day on, William left me strictly alone.

The experience, as I thought about it, brought a dawning realization that strength lies not only in muscles, but in feelings. When my fear gave way to outrage, I was able to scare off a bully who was much bigger than I. Perhaps my stepfather's prescription of two-for-one was the trigger that empowered me.

On the other side of the ledger, I made several close friends in school. I am thinking particularly of Dan, a tallish black boy who walked with two canes and a conspicuous limp long after I was on one brace and one cane. Dan and I liked to play games and hold long talks with each other. On quite a number of occasions I brought him home with me, and my mother treated him as a welcome guest.

I was shocked, therefore, when my mother took me aside one day and told me I mustn't have Dan in the apartment any more, though I could still play with him outside on the street. She explained that other tenants were saying that they didn't like my bringing a black boy into the house.

I was extremely humiliated and didn't know how to break this news to Dan. But he took it in his usual gentle way. We continued to meet on my block, where we played and talked to our heart's content. I tried to pick places where we would be as inconspicuous as possible—not because Dan was black, but because he was lame. As nearly as I can articulate my childhood feelings now, I must have felt that the sight of two lame kids playing together tagged us as creatures of a lower social order. And I had to own up to myself that I felt a curious relief from the pressure of prejudice when our relationship thinned out and finally dissolved. Did I, unconsciously and subliminally, get that shameful message across to Dan?

Mixed in with my relief was a gnawing sense of debasement that I could not yet analyze. Looking back as a therapist, however, I can see that emotionally I identified with Dan. Had I not experienced similar discrimination and rejection because of my body? Dan, being both lame and black, must be experiencing a double dose of prejudice.

I made a promise to myself that someday I was going to do all I could to fight discrimination and help its victims cope. I have kept that promise.

My shining inspiration in those days was Miss Lee, the soft-spoken young teacher who brightened our school days with her constant individual attention and understanding. She was soon curious about my reading, which was not the usual kind. I would talk to her about Goethe's *Faust*, Dante's *Divine Comedy*, Homer's *Odyssey*, and the plays of Euripides.

In our small class there was a great deal of one-on-one instruction, both from the teacher and from some of the older children. Miss Lee used this circumstance to give me a generous amount of her personal attention. She would pull a chair over to my desk and, leaning close to me, go over our lessons. The accidental touch of her hair against my cheek would send me into a golden cloud. Motivated by her constant help and encouragement, I skipped four terms and graduated at the age of twelve instead of fourteen.

Looking back, I would say I was in love with her by a child's standard—certainly not in any amorous way, but in a way that made me feel wonderful just to be close to her. I can also say that the memory of her love and interest in me has been a source of strength through all of my life. She made me feel great.

Toward the end of my last term, our class for "crippled children" was invited to visit the class for "blind children," which was run on much the same basis as ours; that is, all the grades were taught in one room by a single teacher.

I was surprised to find a group of happy kids who behaved much like any other kids. I guess I expected to see children who looked miserable as they groped through their life. I promptly made friends with a nice girl about my own age, and we had a marvelous time comparing notes on what we could and couldn't do. She explained that she could make out shadowy shapes that helped her to find her way and to face the people she was talking to. She relied on sounds, too.

She was very curious about me: How did it feel to be lame? Was it safe for me to cross streets? Did I go to parties? Could I walk in the woods? On my part I wanted to know if she could judge whether she liked a person's face simply by hearing his voice. She told me she could make some good guesses, but she couldn't be sure until she ran her fingers over the face.

"Make a guess about me," I said.

"Well, you have nice eyes, and I would say you're very nice-looking." Then she let her fingers glide gently all over my face and concluded, "My fingers tell me that I can trust you."

By the time our visit was over, I had some very good feelings about her, about myself, and about handicapped people in general. I think it was because I understood that she had learned to accept the way she was and that this was enabling her to accept the way I was. We were two individuals with entirely different handicaps, but each of us was able to reach out and understand the other in terms of his or her own limitations. We connected. We could be friends.

Are handicapped people any less likely to discriminate against people who belong to other types of minorities? I wish I could answer that with a strong affirmative. But I was soon to learn otherwise.

A few days after the term ended, I paid a visit to Andy, a classmate who lived in the Bronx, about five miles from my home. After my friendship with Dan had cooled off, Andy became my buddy and confidant. On this day I spent the last nickel in my pocket to take the subway to his place. When I arrived, I told him I would have to borrow a nickel to get home.

In the middle of a friendly conversation, we somehow got into an argument. I have no idea now what it was about, but it soon got very heated. At the height of the argument, Andy put his mouth close to my ear and dumbfounded me by whispering, "Dirty Jew!"

It was a hammer blow. I was betrayed and stigmatized by my best friend. My old, original shame, unknowingly planted in me by my father in his poetic autobiography, came gushing up under a new name. I suddenly realized that I carried a double stigma—like Dan.

The shame I felt was momentary. Miss Lee had fortified my sense of worth, and my dismay almost instantly turned to anger. I slipped my jacket on and headed for the front door. Andy followed me.

"You need carfare," he said, reaching into his pocket.

I paid no attention to him. I didn't even look around. I simply went out through the front door and began the long trek home. Half way there my feet began to burn, but somehow I made it. I have never seen nor heard from Andy since that day.

———————

TO PARENTS AND OTHER CONCERNED ADULTS: Like most kids, the handicapped child looks to his parents or other significant adults as his role models. If those adults belong to the so-called normal society, he would like to feel that he also belongs in that world.

If he has demonstrated that he can make out well in a class for the able-bodied, and his parents then put him into a class for the physically handicapped, he may interpret this as a failure on his part and label himself as a flawed human being.

If, on the other hand, his disability is so serious that he is bound to suffer isolation in a normal class, the special class can be an enormous boon. Like the therapy groups so popular today, it can offer emotional support, understanding, and encouragement to share his feelings with people who understand.

Perhaps the most important contribution a group can offer a handicapped person is the feeling that "I am not alone." The blind children I met in the school I attended certainly benefited from the program tailored for them and from having a specially trained teacher. The same can hold true for children who are mentally disabled.

If the child is on the borderline of normalcy, this can constitute a serious problem for the concerned parents. Certainly the child's wishes should be consulted and the severity of his handicap appraised. This may call for consultation with a family doctor or a specialist.

My parents must have faced a difficult decision when they overruled my objections to being taken out of a regular public school setting. Though I would say that my mother was definitely overprotective, I can't say that she made the wrong decision in this case.

The possibility of fire, the inevitable stairs, the rushing about of children—all these factors certainly put me at risk.

But it's quite possible that another set of parents would have encouraged me to find my own way, even in the world of the able-bodied. Years and years later I have learned that judgments are dangerous.

What I'm saying again here is that the child's wishes should be respected, but in his own interest they must sometimes be overruled. When they are, a complete explanation should be given. And if the child comes up with convincing reasons to back up his objections, they should be carefully weighed. It might even be a good idea to get some outside opinions.

If you do decide that you must overrule the child for his own sake, make sure you constantly reassure him that you are on his side and ready to listen to him at any time. I have no regrets about being put into Miss Lee's class. That was an extraordinary stroke of luck. But even her loving attention failed to prepare me for the rough demands of the boys' high school that I was later to attend.

As to my parents' decision to bar Dan from our home, that is another serious matter. I feel quite sure that this did not originate with my mother; all her life she was a champion of the black cause, and she taught me by example not to judge people by their color, race, sex, or religion. In the latter part of her life she taught at an all-black high school in Harlem. I suspect that Dan's banishment was largely due to my stepfather, who, without any malice, shared many of the prejudices of his day.

My stepfather—and many other adults—apparently failed to understand that when you reject a member of *any* minority, you are telling the handicapped child subliminally that he, too, is subject to rejection. As a defense, he may even join you in your prejudice as an effort to convince himself that *his* kind of difference is acceptable.

So if you really want to help the handicapped child, your best way of dealing with his fear of rejection is to work on your own prejudices. If you don't want to do that, at least hold them in check when you are around the children.

Another point: When you place your child in a new environment among strangers, make sure you learn how he feels about it. The handicapped child in particular may have some grave misgivings about being put into danger or, worse yet, isolation. He may also feel that you are doing this because he is unworthy.

In a comfortable setting, gently question him about his fears, his frustrations, and his fantasies. When you learn about his feelings, you might do well to question yourself: Are you an overanxious teacher or an overprotective mother? Are the child's feelings unreasonable? Can you let him do what he wants to do without jeopardizing his safety?

When you have fully appraised your child's capabilities and your own fears of giving him more leeway, show your respect for him by acting, as far as possible, on what he tells you. Explain to him that you would like to grant *all* his wishes, but that there are some you can't, since you are responsible for his health and safety, as well as his happiness. But also impress on him that you are willing to discuss his feeling—and yours—at any time and even to change your mind when you are convinced that he's got a case.

Even more important than showing your interest and concern for the child with a disability is helping him to define his own boundaries, and then to come to terms with them.

Many handicapped children have a strong streak of denial; that is, they may refuse to admit to others, or to themselves, that they can't do everything an able-bodied child can do.

Counter this by helping him to discover his own abilities and make the most of them.

CHAPTER
8

THE LITTLE LAME PRINCE

All through my long childhood years I prayed and hoped and fantasized. I have vivid recollections of the make-believes I wove in bed at night. I could picture myself waking up in the morning to find my body miraculously healed. Then I could see myself ice-skating gracefully to the applause of a crowd; or I was dancing on a stage; or I was playing tennis at Wimbleton—on and on. What handicapped child has not regaled himself with fantasies like these?

Sometimes I couldn't resist trying to act out my fantasies. At age eight or nine I was dazzled by a movie version of *The Three Musketeers,* with Douglas Fairbanks, Sr., playing d'Artagnan, the swaggering hero who was always ready for a duel.

On coming home, I swaggered around our apartment, dueling with imaginary opponents. At one point I tried some Fairbanks acrobatics; standing precariously on a chair, I grasped the molding above the double doors between the master bedroom and the living room, and started to swing. Down came the molding, d'Artagnan, and all.

I expected a scolding, but when I looked around, my mother and my brother Ralph were laughing their heads off.

Much of my fantasy life was centered around music. A favorite piece of furniture in our living room was a mahogany Victrola, with a turntable for 78-rpm records on top and a copious cabinet for the disks underneath. I often sat on the floor for an hour or two, playing my favorite recordings. The one I liked best was a Caruso performance of his most famous aria from *Pagliacci*. No matter how many times I played it, that remarkable tenor voice never failed to send streams of energy up and down my body. It would come back to me in bed at night, creating a magic aura around me. Looking back as a therapist, I think what really got to my gut was the sense that Caruso was letting out every little bit of himself without any restraint. I wished with all my might that I could do the same!

But I also had another kind of fantasy, a more beautiful one, stimulated by a children's book my mother had bought for me. It was titled *The Little Lame Prince*. I was quick to identify with him, imagining that I was the prince.

The Little Lame Prince (me) lived a lonely life in the tower of a castle. Because he was lame and lonely, he was chosen to receive a special gift—not from his parents, but from a heavenly, compassionate being. One day this beautiful being brought him a magic carpet. Whenever he wanted to, she explained, the little prince could command his carpet to take him through the skies to any destination he named.

With a gift like that, who would want to be healed? Though part of me knew that this was only make-believe, another part of me was beginning to feel that being lame was actually O.K. In fact, it was great!

As a psychotherapist I have come to appreciate the allegoric significance of the prince's story: My handicap qualified me for inward travel of a kind that helped me in a special way to shape my outer life.

As I grew a little older, perhaps to eleven or twelve, my fantasies began to take a more artistic turn. My mother's record collection had always thrilled me, but now I began going to live concerts. I discovered the Goldman Band, which gave free concerts on the Mall in Central Park. Right after supper I would hurry out to be sure of a front-row seat for the concert. Sometimes my brother Ralph would go with me.

The program usually featured spirited renditions of such classic favorites as the Overture to *Tannhäuser* and the *Ride of the Valkyries,* along with marches by Sousa and by Goldman himself. Caught up in the music, which I came to know by heart, I presently became conscious that my head was bobbing and weaving while I listened in complete rapture.

Soon, however, my mother was taking me rather regularly to Carnegie Hall to hear the world-famous New York Philharmonic orchestra playing under the most renowned conductors. I quickly began to discriminate between Goldman and Toscanini, and the sound quality of the brass band versus the richness of a full orchestra. I became enamored of the Philharmonic and began to picture myself on the podium.

On Sunday afternoons, all through the concert season, the Philharmonic performances were broadcast, and I made sure to tune in on them. Whenever I was safely alone, I would stand up in the living room and "conduct" the music I knew—so vigorously that I would work myself into a happy sweat.

On several occasions my secret performances were so

energetic that I would lose my balance and fall to the floor. Those spills had a dampening effect on me—or you might call it a salutary effect: They made me realize that I could never in this life be an orchestral maestro—at least, not one like Toscanini.

We had a big old upright piano at home, and I tried desperately to play the great works of Wagner, Beethoven, Chopin, and Brahms. On one occasion I heard—and saw— Rachmaninoff perform a concerto with my beloved Philharmonic. This immediately gave birth to a new fantasy—coming on stage, acknowledging the applause, sitting down at the piano and playing thunderously—or dreamily, as the music warranted. But I presently began to doubt that I could ever become a great pianist either.

My thoughtful, pragmatic stepfather had realized this long before I did and had been suggesting that I take up the cello. The cello can be played sitting down, and unlike the piano it requires no footwork. Incidentally, Daddy S. had also urged me to study law so that I might become a judge, another sedentary occupation. I think I finally went him one better: I became an editor, and then a psychotherapist.

———

TO PARENTS AND SURROGATES: It has been observed, both by me and by others, that children who feel isolated and have low self-esteem because of a handicap or poverty or membership in a minority group are more likely to have a rich, magical fantasy life than their mainstream or able-bodied playmates and classmates.

The popular child may tell you of fantasies right in line with his realistic ambitions. He may see himself as a football star or a movie hero. The child who feels isolated by a handicap tends more toward grandiose fantasies that go far beyond what we call reality. The more you examine these observations, the deeper they take you. But the more immediate question here is, what can you do about it to help your child?

Discouraging his fantasies is attacking his problem from the wrong end. Consider, without scoffing, the possibility that his otherworld visitors just might be real entities who are responding to his need. Instead of discounting them, do whatever you can to escalate your child's self-esteem.

Starting with yourself and your family, demonstrate your acceptance and approval in as many ways as you can. Include him in your conversations, your outings, your parties. When feasible, give him your exclusive attention by taking him shopping or out to a ball game. Arrange for him to meet other kids and devise group activities in which he can participate. More than most, the handicapped child needs good parenting.

Fantasies are a way of sorting out the coulds and the couldn'ts. They can have a powerful influence on the way your child lives his life. Children, and grown-ups who have preserved the talent, sooner or later learn to recognize this.

Early in life your child may feel free to talk to you about his inner world. Assume that this is a request for your help in finding out who he is. If he tells you that he killed a wicked ogre and rescued a beautiful princess, just comment on the great love he must feel for that princess if he is willing to risk his life for her. In other words, dwell on the positive aspect.

The "reality" of fantasies is attested to by the powerful influence they can have on an individual's direction in life. Instead of dismissing them wholesale, you can help your child to discover which fantasies are destructive and which will contribute to his growth.

With this in mind, the most helpful response you can make when your child opens up his fantasy world to you is to join him in that world. Ask questions, collaborate with him, become his secret ally. Ask him where his magic carpet is taking him, and present your own opinions. In this way you can offer guidance.

If you can collaborate with your child in this manner, you have a very effective strategy for instilling your own values in him.

CHAPTER
9

MY BIG BROTHER AND ME

Of all my relatives and friends, the one person I was really closest to throughout my growing years was my brother Ralph. He was a delicate-looking boy with wavy black hair, a handsome face, and a shy manner. His main ambition, at least most of the time, was to be a playwright. Though he was four years older than I, he always treated me as an equal—even when I was very little. While he understood my physical limitations, he was far more interested in my abilities, both physical and mental.

Together we wrote plays and stories, and invented gadgets that didn't work too well. In the old-fashioned boarding house in the Poconos, where our family usually spent the summer, there was a large "parlor," as they called it; here boarders and wandering entertainers could display their talents. Ralph and I liked to put on a variety show, for which we enlisted other children to dance and sing or take part in the playlets that Ralph and I (mostly Ralph) scripted.

The feature of the evening was always a magic show, performed by "Oppenheim the Great" before our very charitable audience. I was perhaps nine or ten years old at the time. Ralph and I would work out the script and the tricks together, injecting as much patter as we could to divert the audience's attention from my sleight of hand. A sad sample of our patter:

> While traveling on business, two brothers named Timmy and Jimmy stopped at a hotel on a warm night. Before going to bed they tried to open the window to let in some air, but the window was stuck. Finally they went to bed anyway, but they couldn't sleep. They kept complaining to each other that the heat was more than they could stand.
>
> Finally Timmy got an idea. "Let's throw one of your shoes at the window so we don't die of the heat."
>
> Jimmy thought that was a great idea. He immediately picked up a heavy shoe and gave it to Timmy to throw. Timmy put all his might into the pitch. The brothers heard the glass shattering in the dark, and after a few moments they could feel the cool air flowing in.
>
> "Ah, that feels good!" Jimmy said with a sigh of relief. Timmy agreed, and soon the brothers fell sound asleep.
>
> Next morning Timmy was the first to wake up. "Jimmy!" he called out, "Take a look!"
>
> The glass windowpane was intact, but a mirror on the wall beside it was shattered.

The laughter in the audience may have been rather forced, but at the time it sounded to me like an ovation. More important, this fictive anecdote constituted an important step for me: It was my first attempt to give expression to a principle I had already discovered by myself: namely, that mind can be more powerful than matter. It's the same principle that doctors recognized long ago when they gave out those little pink sugar pills. They called them placebos.

Bloated with success, I went back to school in the fall and offered to put on my magic show for the class. Miss Lee, our ever-permissive teacher, gave me the go-ahead. My classmates, however, were not as charitable as the adult audience where I premiered my show. The kids saw right through most of my tricks and had no hesitation in calling my bluffs on the spot.

The experience disillusioned me about the kudos I had gathered in my summer performance. It made me realize that all the applause and praise were motivated by a desire to make the little lame boy feel good.

Ralph and I were always giving each other ideas to bring glory or money to us. My unpredictable mother was surprisingly tolerant of some and surprisingly forbidding about others for reasons that we could never fathom. While we were in the Poconos, she allowed us to go into business with a children's photo-finishing set; it lasted about a week. When one of our first customers, a nice, elderly lady, showed us some commercial prints she'd had made, from the same negatives Ralph and I had processed for her, we had to acknowledge that our prints were pale by comparison. We sadly refunded her money and gave up the business. But that didn't stop us from trying; we never seemed to be without ideas.

Back in New York we acquired a hectograph, which is a tray filled with a kind of gelatinous stuff that can take the impression of a typed page. This can be used as a negative to make positive prints. The resultant copy was purple and fuzzy. We promptly got out a newspaper and went to Riverside Park to sell it for a nickel a copy.

Our first customer was a very pleasant man, who gave us a nickel for his paper and complimented us both on our enterprising spirit. But right at that point, our angry mother swooped down on us, demanding to know what was going on. When she found out that we had launched a business behind her back, she ordered us to give the nickel back to our customer.

That good man, seeing our embarrassment, said, "Why don't you let them make this one sale?" But Mom was adamant.

One day Ralph came home from attending a perfor-mance of Ibsen's *Peer Gynt* with our mother. That evening he told me all about the trolls—repulsive underground creatures that you wouldn't want to meet on a moonless night. We decided that the word applied to many of the people we knew and that the world's population was di-vided into trolls and nontrolls.

We defined nontrolls as the spiritual people who feel that we are watched over by beings from another realm, people who express their feelings in poetry and fine fiction, in painting and sculpture and dancing, as well as in sensitive responses to other nontrolls. I am using terminology that we were not yet educated enough to utilize at the time; but we relied on our own judgment to distinguish the nontrolls from the far more numerous trolls.

In our opinion (and please remember that we presently grew out of this childish snobbery), trolls, basically, are materialistic. They build their lives around money and pos-sessions instead of art, love, and spiritual development. If our definitions were applied today, they would include people who have no regard for the environment, who are more interested in profit than in the gifts our planet provides.

We soon added a special category of trolls: nice trolls. These were friendly, generous people who just were not in touch with the Higher Power. We decided that Daddy S. was a nice troll, while Daddy O. was definitely a nontroll. I don't think we ever got around to classifying our mother. Looking back from today's vantage point, I think we would have called her a stormy nontroll.

When either of us was away from home, we wrote long letters to each other, setting forth our theories and pigeonholing all the people we knew. Along with each letter we sent home, we'd be sure to enclose a "Mother letter," filled with all the banalities we could think of. This was for self-protection, so that we could always have a letter to show Mom. We kept the important letters in a secret file.

Ralph and I, of course, rated ourselves as way up in the higher echelons of nontrolls. In short, we were snobs—snobs of a special kind. We felt that our sense of connection with the Higher Power put us a cut above most of the people around us.

We had a secret meeting place, where we would converse with the spirits. In Riverside Park, near 83rd Street there is a huge rock in the shape of a mound. It's known as Mount Tom. It was not difficult for me to climb to the top, which was a good place for many kids, including us, to fly their kites.

Ralph and I had discovered a hidden entrance to a cave, deep down in the bowels of Mount Tom, and we would go there at midnight, while our parents and brother Louis were sleeping. There we would call up the spirits and ask them for advice on such problems as how to handle ourselves when Mom was quarreling with Daddy S., or for ideas on our writing projects. In the morning, we would discuss whatever the spirits had told us.

Sometimes we would encounter frightening creatures in the cave. Then we had to hide in the crannies until we could make our escape. This lent a feeling of excitement and suspense to our visits, which were always top secret. We never

told Mom or Daddy S., or even Daddy O. about these midnight adventures.

There is no cave in Mount Tom. At least that's what the
trolls would tell you. Ralph and I made our midnight visits
without our earthly bodies ever leaving our beds. It was all
pretty real to us. And pretty nice. It expanded our egos to
know that we had a secret territory that was all our own, to
govern as we wished.

Another enticing road to the world of magic and even to
the realm of metaphysics was the Ouija board, which enjoyed a brief craze among the people we knew. As soon as I
heard about this promising way of communicating with the
spirits, I knew I had to have a Ouija board.

If you are not familiar with the Ouija board, let me explain it. It's a smooth board, small enough to hold on your
lap. In the upper corners are the words yes and no. The al-
phabet is stamped in an arc across the board. It comes with
a small, triangular piece of wood or plastic, called a
planchette, that has three little legs, each tipped with felt so
that it glides easily across the smooth board.

The operator places his hand lightly on the planchette,
asks the spirit a question and waits for the planchette to
move around the board without any guidance from him. In
this manner, the spirit can answer questions with yes or no,
or can spell out answers by moving from letter to letter. That
is the theory behind the board, and it seems that two persons facing each other are likely to get better results than a
single operator.

Many individuals who have true psychic ability advise
against the use of Ouija boards. They will tell you that the
Ouija board can be extremely dangerous for anybody who
has no expertise in dealing with spirits. For one thing, they
say that you never know what spirits will respond to you.
You may call in negative entities who give misleading infor-

mation that can put you in harm's way. But these caveats had not reached me at that time.

I tried the Ouija board with many of my friends who were willing and watched them try it among themselves. The results I obtained by myself or with partners were highly questionable. The planchette would move hesitantly, going to letters that didn't spell anything. I had to strain my sense of plausibility to imagine I was in touch with the spirit world.

Finally I asked my brother Ralph to try it with me on the premise that the extraordinary spiritual affinity between us might produce a result.

We sat opposite each other in my bedroom with the Ouija board between us and called out, "Are you there?" Then we waited expectantly for the planchette to move. It did, eventually, but with hesitation and apparent lack of purpose. As usual, it went to letters that didn't spell anything we could fathom. We kept repeating, "Are you there?"

Suddenly the planchette took off, so fast that our hands had trouble keeping up with it. I looked at Ralph accusingly and said, "You did that!" He swore innocence and replied that he had the same feeling about me. So we addressed the presumed spirit:

"Who are you?"

The planchette swiftly spelled out "Bob Hatfield." By now it was clear that neither of us was influencing the movement of the planchette. So we pushed on with our questioning. Bob Hatfield volunteered, "I knew your father."

Further questioning established that he was referring to Daddy O., who had passed on by this time, and that Bob Hatfield was himself a poet, which made sense.

I asked him, "Have any of your poems been published?"

Instead of going to the Yes at an upper corner of the board, the planchette took a shortcut and landed on the letter S.

I said, "I haven't seen any of your poems. Have you ever published a book?"

"S."

"Do we have your book?"

There was a brief pause, and then, "S."

"Is it in this room?"

"S."

"Where is it?"

"Bookcase next to your bed," the planchette spelled out.

"Which shelf?" I asked.

"Second shelf. Green book on right side."

I went over to the bookcase and pulled out a slender green book. Ralph still had his fingers on the planchette, so I asked, "This one?"

"S."

I said, "This is a book of poetry by Stephen Spender. It's not yours."

There was another pause. Then the planchette spelled out, "Sorry, I thought it was."

At this point we heard our mother calling us for dinner. Ralph said, "We have to go for supper now. Will you be here when we get back?"

"S."

As soon as dinner was over, Ralph and I hurried back to the Ouija board. I asked, "Are you still there, Bob?"

"S," the planchette responded without the slightest hesitation.

"Have you anything important to say to us?" I ventured, and the answer came right back:

"Seek your father in the gray land."

Ralph and I looked at each other in utter bewilderment. For some reason I found myself associating the gray land with a phrase used by Carl Jung, the great Swiss psychiatrist whose personal influence had turned my father's whole life around. More recently Daddy O. had written to him for help in a period of deep distress, and Jung had replied: "I advise you to look within."

I had always looked on such advice, whether from psychics or psychiatrists or entities from the other side, as a strategy for putting the ball right back in the questioner's court. Years later, when I became more familiar with the work of Edgar Cayce, the well-known psychic of the first half of the 20th century, and the metaphysical writings of such literary giants as William Blake, Plato, Aldous Huxley, William Butler Yeats, et al, I began to perceive the meaning of the "gray land" or "looking within." Both phrases, as I understand them, refer to the inner mind, or what is commonly called the unconscious. In that gray land, I believe, is all the wisdom we need to take charge of our life. In one way or another, that is what I tell my patients today. I like to think of it as the inner mind.

At that time, however, neither Ralph nor I could make anything out of the message on the Ouija board. Perhaps our spirit guest sensed this. From there on we got very little—just the kind of jumbled responses I had experienced with my friends.

It certainly seemed to both Ralph and me that the planchette had moved without any direction from our hands. Was that an illusion? Was it some mischievous spirit playing games with us? Was it truly the spirit of Bob Hatfield? Or was it a kind of energy that grew out of my rapport with my brother? Why could we never find any book of poems by Bob Hatfield? Was this because they may have been privately printed?

In sum, our experiment escalated my resolve to pursue my quest—but without benefit of the Ouija board.

————————

TO PARENTS AND SURROGATES: A good precept to keep in mind is that your child's fantasies are real to him.

Another good precept is that they should be accepted, and even encouraged, so long as they are not frightening to the child.

When your little boy tells you that a beautiful woman with blue wings visits him every night and holds his hand while she sings him to sleep, don't just smile. Tell him how wonderful that is. Ask him: "What does she wear? What kind of songs does she sing? Does she ever talk? How long does she stay?" In short, draw the child out by showing your interest.

Remember that children are generally quick to perceive the way grown-ups feel. A tolerant smile on your face may be an instant signal for your child to clam up. In my own case, I knew that my Daddy S. was a nonbeliever, and that Daddy O., while he never scoffed, listened with the ears of a psychoanalyst. I think that Mom was the one who felt the reality of my stories—but only at times; she was unpredictable. Given this kind of audience, Ralph and I learned, as children, to keep our otherworld experiences to ourselves.

As I look back on the fantasies we generated, singly or in collaboration, I would say that some of them were good for us and some were not. Our whole concept of a world populated by trolls and nontrolls was not conducive to happy relationships. It was like saying that people are either bad or good. And as the good guys, we were fostering an unhealthy kind of snobbery.

From my own experiences as a child and later as a therapist, I would advise parents to help the child sort out his fantasies or contacts with otherworld spirits. It might have made my own life more comfortable if my parents had pointed out that all people have goodness in them; and rather than pinning labels on a person, it would be more helpful all around to look for the good qualities, and then tell that person how much you appreciate them.

On the other hand, if your child is seeking contact with

spirits, largely for the purpose of astonishing his friends, it might mean that he is suffering from a terrible sense of aloneness or unworthiness and a need for approval.

But it also might have another, far more significant meaning: Perhaps your child is really in touch with a world beyond our ken. Please, don't ever, ever scoff!

CHAPTER
10

MY LITTLE BROTHER AND ME

I was four years old when my half-brother Louis (rhymes with Dewey) was born. While he was in his infancy, Ralph and I got fed up with our parents' pride and love for him. We would go around the apartment chanting:

> Louis, Louis,
> What did you dooey?
> PYOOEY!

Daddy S. didn't like that little poem. He said we shouldn't talk that way about our baby brother, and he suggested that we make up a rhyme starting, "How we love our brother Louis!" Somehow we never got around to that.

I think this was the beginning of my serious troubles at home. Looking back, I feel sure that Daddy S. never played favorites—surely not wittingly—but at that time Ralph and

I *felt* that he did. The feeling didn't stop me from loving my little brother and doing all kinds of things with and for him. As we grew up, Lou and I slept in a double-decker bed where we could talk in whispers and plot our latest mischief.

Many years later I learned that Louis had always felt sort of out of it, because Ralph and I had a glamorous writer for a father and could talk literary language. He didn't know that I was also feeling out of it, because Lou was physically so enviable—a swimmer, a runner, a hiker, a Boy Scout leader and definitely his parents' favorite, a position I had once felt secure in.

Lou and I went canoeing and hiking together, to the extent of my abilities. We went to summer camp together. And though we would each hang out with kids our own age, we were always close to each other.

It was Lou who introduced me to the magic of hypnosis. One of the adult counselors had given him some coaching in the art, and Lou was quick to make it into a fun thing. He hypnotized one camper and got him to pursue another camper right down to the lake, where the fugitive jumped in, clothes and all. Everybody thought that was sensational.

A summer or so later, Lou and I and two school friends were camping by a lake in Pennsylvania where, in those days, you had to pitch a tent if you wanted shelter from the weather. In a nearby tent was a gang of tough-looking teenagers—from Scranton, Pennsylvania, as we soon learned. They looked like street kids, the kind we had no desire to tangle with.

One of the boys from our tent, while talking to the Scranton boys, boasted that we had a hypnotist in our group.

"Oh yeah?" was the cynical reaction. "Why don't you show us?"

"Sure, we'll show you. Why don't you come over to our campfire tonight?"

The invitation was accepted, and my brother spent the day in anxious anticipation. Those Scranton kids didn't look like ideal subjects for hypnosis.

Night came. We built the campfire, and we waited. My brother paled a little when he saw the Scranton troop approaching. Without any of the usual amenities, one of the Scrantonites pointed to the biggest, meanest-looking guy in their group and said, "Here's your man."

I thought my brother was about to pass out, but he pulled himself together and invited his subject into our tent, telling him to lie down on a cot. Lou seated himself next to the cot and was about to start a hypnotic induction. But before he could get a word out of his mouth, he could see that his subject was in deep, deep trance.

Lou told the Scrantonite to get up and guided him out to the wide-eyed group around the campfire. He handed his man a lemon and told him it was a delicious candy. The Scrantonite took it eagerly and ate the whole lemon, skin, pits, and all. The audience gasped.

Next, my brother told his subject that his arms couldn't feel anything. Then he sterilized a needle with a match and ran it right through the fleshy biceps. There was not a wince from the hypnotized giant.

My brother said, "I'm going to count to three and snap my fingers. As soon as I snap my fingers you'll wake up." And so saying, Lou counted and snapped his fingers.

The big tough guy from Scranton immediately fell forward, flat on his stomach, face down, with his hair about four inches from the campfire. At this, my brother really did turn white. He got down on the ground and promptly put his subject back into hypnosis, assuring him that when he woke up he would feel fine and have no memory of his trance experience.

By rare good fortune the Scrantonite was one of those one-in-a-hundred people capable of immediate somnambulism, as the deepest level of hypnosis is called, and the situation ended gloriously for my brother.

Watching all the proceedings, I was emotionally shaken up, both by this dramatic demonstration of the extraordinary power of hypnosis and of the grave dangers of using it without knowing what you're doing. I decided then and there not to fool around with it until I was thoroughly trained. Many years later, hypnosis was to become my chief tool as a therapist.

———

TO PARENTS AND STEPPARENTS: Sibling rivalry is said to exist in practically every family with more than one child. Most parents these days have a pretty good understanding of it. However, when a handicapped boy or girl is confronted with a new brother or sister, and sees—or imagines he sees—favoritism, he will very likely blame it on his impaired body.

He may make painstaking observations of his mother's pleasure in playing with the baby's feet and remarking on the newcomer's beautiful little body. He may see the joyful relationship between father and baby. No matter how hard his parents try to avoid playing favorites or how well they succeed, the handicapped child may be nursing a secret grievance because the baby has all his limbs intact, while he himself does not.

As a parent, you have been tossed a difficult job—one that calls for sensitivity and lots of love. But it is a challenge you can meet. Here are some thoughts:

Emphasize to the handicapped child how important he's going to be in his little brother's life; how much he has to teach this newcomer—like drawing pictures for him or showing him how mechanical toys work; what fun it's going to be to have someone to play with, to share his secrets with; how he can set an example that will help his baby brother grow into a beautiful person, and how that little brother is going to love him for the rest of his life.

As the new baby grows into an able child, plan as many activities as you can in which both children can participate. Car trips, movies, carefully chosen games—these are good examples you might start with. And when friends or strangers rave about the beautiful baby, introduce him, not as "my latest," but as "Jimmy's new brother." When taking family snapshots, try to include some pictures of Jimmy holding the baby.

It's often best to leave the question of the older brother's handicap alone; let the children work it out in their own way. When the little one starts asking his brother about it, chances are he'll get honest answers that will strengthen the bond between them.

CHAPTER
11

LEARNING MY BOUNDARIES

"A lake is something limited. Water is inexhaustible. A lake can contain only a definite amount of the infinite quantity of water . . . In human life, too, the individual achieves significance through discrimination and the setting of limits . . . Unlimited possibilities are not suited to man; if they existed, his life would only dissolve in the boundless . . . The individual attains significance as a free spirit only by surrounding himself with these limitations."
I Ching (roughly translated)

All through my grammar-school years in the warm, sheltered environment created by Miss Lee in her special class, I could dream myself into grandeur without hindrance. I could hardly wait to get out into the wider world and make these dreams come true.

When I graduated from elementary school at the age of twelve, my mother wanted to enroll me in the Ethical Culture school, a fine institution practicing some advanced ideas to encourage their students to blossom. We paid a visit to John Lovejoy Elliot, the school's director. This fatherly philosopher explained to us that I would have to start in the eighth grade, which I had already completed in public school, so as to be prepared for his school's unique approach. That would have meant putting off my entrance into the grown-up world for five years.

I held out for Townsend Harris Hall, a high school for bright boys that condensed the standard four-year program into three. It was financed by the City of New York and affiliated with City College, on whose campus it stood.

Three years against five? For this impatient boy there was no choice. I nagged with all my might, and this time, as often, I had my way.

Coming from Miss Lee's class, where tending the goldfish and the plants was just as important as learning about the verbs and adjectives, I was soon lost in a bleak, competitive atmosphere among all the bright boys. I realized that virtually all sports were out of my reach and that I was not eligible for membership in some clubs, such as the ones for students interested in hiking or social dancing. I did what I could, however, editing the class paper, participating in the debating society, and trying to bring my fantasies more in line with the new realities I now faced.

No more buses to pick me up and deliver me; I lugged my books to school by subway now, and it was a walk at both ends. The few handicapped students in the school were allowed to use the elevator to reach their classrooms, but "leaving the room" entailed a trip to the basement—and the elevator operator was hardly ever available between periods. I readily adapted to these physical demands.

As to scholarship, I felt sure that my extensive background in the classics would enable me to breeze through. I chose Latin over French as my primary language and opted for Greek as the second one. I did well in Greek, as I was already versed in that country's mythology. But there was a problem: Every class was required to have a minimum enrollment of six students, and we had just five.

The problem was solved when my civics teacher joined the class as the sixth student. At term's end, however, we learned that he had failed the course, and that the class was being discontinued.

I was at the top of the class in English, without ever doing my homework, and I enjoyed special after-class chats with two of my English teachers who took a kindly interest in me.

I keenly disliked a certain mathematics instructor, and I tried to cover up my feelings by cracking jokes in his class. Everybody laughed except Mr. Smith, the teacher. He reprimanded me several times for being disruptive, but I went right on joking. The words just seemed to issue from my mouth without any intention on my part.

The passing grade was 65, and at the end of the term, when the final marks were posted, I was shocked to see that mine was 64. Hardly believing what I saw, I went upstairs into the math teacher's classroom and asked why he could not allow me that one little extra point that would keep me from flunking.

"I'll tell you why," he said, without ever cracking a smile. "You were always disrupting the class with your jokes."

I couldn't muster any answer; I was dumbfounded by this spiteful injustice. Looking back, I wonder why my parents didn't talk to the principal about it when I told them. They just let it go.

I told myself that I really didn't care about marks. I was still daydreaming about the great things I would do when I was free to pursue my career. I could see myself walking onto a stage as Oppenheim the Great Magician, or playing

Tchaikovsky's piano concerto in Carnegie Hall, or dancing with a ballet troupe.

Only there was a difference now: I was beginning to acknowledge to myself that some of my dreams were out of my reach—that I really did have some serious limitations—limitations imposed on me by an accidental exposure to the polio virus.

Or was it really accidental? Later in my life I was to get an astonishing answer to that question.

Meanwhile, I was learning to discriminate between dreams that could never be fulfilled and those ambitions that were within the realm of the possible. I thought of the former as fantasies I could use to promote inner good feelings, and the latter as goals I could choose to set my sights on.

Around this time my superactive mother was taking courses at Teachers College, where she also used the swimming pool. One day she was talking about me to the swimming instructor, Doc Holm, who promptly said, "Bring him around to me."

Doc Holm, a benign, fatherly looking man who exuded goodwill, also taught swimming at Columbia University. I found him standing poolside in his swimsuit, shouting instructions to a class of naked youngsters. He told me to strip in the shower room and come to him after the class was over.

I was both excited and skeptical about what he might do for me. I had always been fascinated by the idea of gliding through the water under my own power, but had classified that daydream as one that was out of my reach.

Doc Holm produced a pair of water wings, which he pumped full of air and then attached to me. "You can't sink while you're wearing these," he explained, "so just jump in."

His words brought an immediate flash of memory into my mind. In the Poconos I had seen a mother bird and her fledgling on the ledge of a building. The little bird was making a big fuss because the mother bird was nudging it to take off from the ledge. The sound was truly pitiful. But finally the mother bird gave her fledgling a push, and the tiny bird was suddenly in mid-air. Its wings began to flap wildly, and a moment later it was flying. Chirping boastfully, it flew in a circle several times, then landed happily on the ledge to receive its mother's congratulations.

With that nudge from my memory bank, I flopped into the water. Next thing I knew, I was enthusiastically taking orders from Doc Holm.

I visited the pool three times a week, and each time Doc Holm put a little less air into the water wings. One day he said, "There's no air in those wings. You're swimming with a dead weight."

Because of the special configuration of residual muscle in my legs, I was able to swim much faster on my back than I could with the crawl or the breast stroke. In fact I put on speed that was almost as great as what the able-bodied students could display.

One day, using a combination of back stroke and crawl, I was able to swim a full mile in the pool while Doc Holm stood at one end and counted the pool lengths for me.

My accomplishments in the pool encouraged me to take my parents' advice and go to a summer camp in the Adirondacks. I soon had a beautiful tan, muscular arms, and a mixed disposition. I liked what the exercise and sunshine were doing for my body. I liked the marshmallow roasts, the amateur theatricals, the meals served at a long table with a laughing crowd, and, most of all, the feeling of belonging.

On the other hand, I felt that somehow all this physical activity might be interfering with the artistic and spiritual life I wanted to lead. As a result, I waffled from enthusiastic participation to self-imposed isolation.

Twice a day I was down at the dock to await the arrival of the pickle boat, as we called it—a little paddle-wheel boat that brought the mail and carried provisions for sale. I was always in suspense as I looked for letters from my Daddy O. in California or my mother in New York. She often sent little packages of fudge and other goodies.

Most of all I was looking for letters from Hannah, a motherly girl I had met the previous summer in the Poconos. I was fifteen at the time, and Hannah was seventeen. Her photograph in soft focus was always on my dresser, at home or at camp. I was hopelessly in love with her, but I'm afraid that she regarded me as just a good friend. The pickle boat rarely brought me the letter I wanted most. When it came, it was always just a friendly letter.

Aside from my secret longing, I was making a lot of friends. I became especially close to one of the counselors. John was blessed with a body that had everything mine lacked: stature, broad shoulders, strong legs, and several athletic skills.

My only athletic skills were swimming and canoeing, but I was pretty good at both. I often went canoeing by myself; it was my way of getting in touch with that Creative Force I was always thinking about. At other times John and I would paddle together and rest together on the little islands that dotted the lakes. We would lie on the ground and talk for hours about camp, girls, our families, our schools, anything.

One of the great accomplishments a camper could achieve was to swim across the lake, a distance of about a mile and a half. Every camper who performed this feat was a hero for a day. Toward the end of the season, I arranged to try it, with my friend John escorting me in a canoe.

It was easier to swim a mile and a half this way than to do a mile in the Columbia pool, where I had to turn around and push off every pool length. My feat was honored by an announcement at dinnertime.

This ego booster was soon counterbalanced by a crusher. One beautiful afternoon, while John and I were canoeing near the shore, we saw two girls in bathing suits sitting on a dock and holding a conversation punctuated by many giggles.

John promptly peeled off his T-shirt and, wearing only his swimsuit, leaped into the lake with a Tarzan-like cry. The next minute he was climbing onto the pier to the welcoming laughter of the two pretty girls.

I was astonished to see that they didn't immediately tell John to go jump back into the lake. How did he know that he would get such a friendly reception? All sorts of feelings and questions swirled within me.

I felt betrayed, envious, helpless, and abandoned by my friend, while at the same time I found myself wishing him luck. But in my secret heart the scene was a clear confirmation of my feeling that I was forever shut out from such happy guy-girl relationships.

And why, you may well ask, didn't I do something about it? Why didn't I just go over and join the happy trio? I was dressed in a one-piece swimsuit and a pair of long pants to hide my undeveloped leg. I had left my brace behind, so I was unable to walk properly. No way could I compete with the superb physique and bold manner of my best friend. Young girls, I told myself, look only at the externals; they are captivated by an athletic body and have no use for a lively mind or a beautiful personality.

How little I knew!

———————

TO CONCERNED ADULTS: The poor man dreams of wealth. The slave dreams of freedom. The rejected lover dreams of total acceptance—or sometimes total power over the beloved. All these fantasies, no matter how far-fetched, are within the realm of the possible. But when the youngster with a permanently impaired body fantasizes physical wholeness, he may be setting himself up for a heartbreaking disenchantment.

As he grows toward adulthood, he begins to sense the difference between real life and fantasy life. Even as a small child, I probably realized that the fantasy of being the Little Lame Prince and having a magic carpet at my disposal was a fairy tale. But this delightful story may have sent a message to my inner mind that my disability could somehow bring me an exceptional gift.

So I would suggest to all concerned adults that telling a disabled youngster, "You can be anything you want to be if you just go for it" may not be very helpful. Suppose this youngster wishes he could be a concert pianist but has only one good leg to operate the three pedals on a concert grand? Ask yourself whether you might not be leading him on by getting him stirred up with an ambition that could bring him to an emotional crash.

On the other hand, telling him, "You can't be a concert pianist without two good feet," while realistic, is not going to make him feel very happy about himself. What's more, it might not even be true.

A better approach, to my mind, is to help him find out whether there isn't some way he can operate the three pedals with one foot. For example, an iron bar can be designed with a clamp on one end to fit over a pedal, and a spring under the other end, where the heel of the good foot can rest. If such an accessory is properly designed, the pianist can train himself to reach all three pedals with ease, using both his heel and his toes. I designed such an accessory and used it, when I was taking piano lessons in my youth.

There are always many ways of tackling a problem. Itzhak Perlman, who walks with the aid of two crutches, didn't let his handicap stop him from becoming one of the world's greatest violinists. When he performs on the concert stage, he plays sitting down.

———

TO HANDICAPPED TEEN-AGERS: A permanent disability is a condition of life that has been handed to you to cope with. If you believe (as I do) that everything that happens happens for a reason, it might be very rewarding for you to speculate on the reason for your handicap. Could it be to strengthen your character? To increase your understanding of other people who must go through life with a disadvantage? To work off a sense of guilt or shame that you brought with you from some previous lifetime?

Somewhere inside of you, in the inner mind—or subconscious, as it is also called—are the answers to these questions. You may seek your own answers by delving inward through meditation or prayer or with the help of an understanding hypnotherapist or psychotherapist. The answers, when you find them, will do much to give meaning and purpose to your life.

CHAPTER
12

GROWING UP

Two unusual objects have graced my bookcase for a long, long time. One is an exquisite fan carved of razor-thin petals of driftwood, spreading upward from a simple pedestal and notched together at the top to form a perfect arc. The other is a tiny cage with four upright posts that imprison a little wooden ball; my friends shake it and ask how the ball ever got into the cage. Each of these objects was carved with a penknife from a single piece of driftwood and in a very few minutes, by a man I'll call Aram. As I say, this was many years ago.

I don't remember exactly how we got to talking with each other. I was coming home from high school on one of those double-decker Fifth Avenue buses that have vanished from the Manhattan scene. A young stranger who was seated beside me was telling me that he was a real Ojibwa Indian. He had come all the way from Canada, he said, to have some fun and make a lot of money in New York. He made money wherever he went, he explained, by doing real Indian dances. In nightclubs. In costume.

"I'm terrific," he confided, and his tone made it sound as if I were the one being flattered.

Aram had short black hair and a handsome, outdoorsy face with deep-set eyes. I sensed that his body, hidden by a jacket much too large for him, had a kind of animal litheness. I could smell it. He may have been dirty, too, now that I come to think of it; but I didn't then—I was only fourteen and a half, though I readily passed for eighteen.

"Why don't we go out together tonight?" Aram suggested. "You can show me some of the hot spots in Greenwich Village. We can meet some girls. We can have some fun."

His black eyes were very close to me, and they dazzled. No adult had ever before treated me so much like an equal. Doors inside of me flew open, revealing a thousand enticing new possibilities. Then they closed.

"I have no money," I said, shamed and stigmatized that so small an obstacle should stand in the way of such an exciting prospect.

Aram drew back and looked me over carefully, from the part in my hair to the shape of my shoes. "Your dad will give it to you," he said. I immediately believed him.

We got off the bus at 83rd Street and Riverside Drive. But instead of going directly to my apartment, we decided, at Aram's suggestion, to take a walk first.

"Let's go down to the river and find some wood," he said. "I'll make you something wonderful that you can keep."

So Aram was going to let me find out right away whether he was the kind of man who delivered on his shiny promises. If he really and truly made me something wonderful, all the other marvels would follow naturally. Or so I reasoned.

The importance of that afternoon is locked in the amber

of my memory. I can see the tall stranger and the curious
adolescent seated together on a weathered wooden beam
near the riverfront, Aram examining the bits of driftwood
he'd collected, testing them for dampness, judging them for
size.

Suddenly he opened his penknife and started whittling
and slicing and gouging. In no time at all he presented me
with the two astonishing little treasures. I thought that the
fan was the most beautiful piece of handicraft I'd ever seen,
and the caged ball was surely the cleverest. Aram shrugged
off my compliments with a wise smile and suggested that
we move along to prepare for the big night ahead of us.

My mother, who thought nothing of bedding down the
strangers my brothers and I were always bringing home,
greeted Aram casually. She exclaimed over his woodcarv-
ing, and when she learned that he had no place to sleep,
promptly offered him my trundle bed for the night.

When Daddy S. came home, Aram volunteered to demonstrate his Indian dance, and we all sat around the living
room while he leaped and postured, shading his eyes with
his hand to peer into the distance. He kept thrusting his
behind out so far, so often, and so abruptly that I couldn't
stop laughing—and wondering if I was being rude.

I told my stepfather I wanted to show Aram some of the
sights of the city but that I was short of funds. He slipped me
a ten-dollar bill, and Aram and I were soon on our way to
the Village.

I suggested that we try the Purple Barn. I'd never been
inside of that establishment, but I'd heard a lot of talk about
it. It was filled with girls accompanied by girls, and men accompanied by men, all obviously interested in sex, one way
or another. I told Aram to take charge of my ten dollars,
since I had no idea of how to tip or when.

Aram picked a table in the center of the room and ordered two beers. He blew some of the head off his, sipped it,

and surveyed the sex-drenched scene with the eyes of an expert. Pretty soon he got up from the table and said, "Watch this."

Two tables away I heard him saying, "I'm an Indian and a stranger in town. I'm looking for a little companionship."

One of the three girls at the table gave him a weary stare and said, "Why don't you just nip over to Macy's? I hear they have a lot of dummies there." Aram moved off with dignity, trailed by mocking laughter.

At the next table he made out better. I saw a very thin girl shrug and make room for him on her bench. He sat down, signaling me to join him. I took our beers over. An attractive, heavily rouged girl opposite Aram's companion moved over to make room for me.

"Hello, Junior, I'm Gladys," my girl said. "You look a little nicer than your friend over there."

"So do you," I said, pleased with my ready wit.

Now our waiter was upon us, protesting that we couldn't change tables because he would lose his tip. Aram put folded money into his hand, and he left us.

Aram ordered a round of drinks, and soon my brains were floating in clouds of alcohol. As my inhibitions dissolved, I began to make cautious advances on Gladys. She drew my hand firmly away. "I'm drinking Scotch," she said. "Be a good boy and order me a double."

I started to signal the waiter, but Aram interrupted me. "Wait," he said. Then, turning to his companion, "We are strangers in town here. You are the hostesses. I think it would be right for you to buy *us* a drink now."

The thin girl got up from the table, "Listen to the Indian giver," she said. "But on second thought, don't listen to him. C'mon, Gladys."

There was barely enough money left to pay the bill, practically nothing for the tip. We left with an angry waiter's assurance that he had a long memory.

I didn't care. I was ecstatic. Aram had made good on everything. He had carved wonderful gifts. We had gone to Greenwich Village, met girls, had fun. I couldn't understand why he seemed so downcast on the subway going home. I would have done anything for him right then. Anything.

Back home, while we were undressing, I learned the reason for Aram's depression. "I have an audition tomorrow," he said. "But no costume. If I can just raise enough money for a costume, I've got a job. Otherwise ... "

Was I really willing to do anything for Aram? I felt an unpleasant pressure mounting inside of me. A secondhand costume, he said, would cost about $25. There was no risk, of course; he could repay it tomorrow night after his new employer gave him an advance on his salary. It was his only chance.

"I don't have that much money," I said apologetically.

"Your dad?"

"He never will. Do you want me to ask him?"

"Never mind." Aram slumped onto the trundle bed, and my guilt expanded. I was thinking of my savings account, which had $37 and some change in it.

"Isn't there anybody else you could borrow from?" I asked.

"You're the only friend I have in New York."

"What happens if you can't get the money?"

Aram shrugged. "Who knows? Breadlines. Jail, maybe."

"Look," I said. "I have a little over $25 in a savings account. Maybe ... "

Aram sat up and grabbed my hand. "I knew you'd be a real friend," he said. "I knew that the minute I laid eyes on you."

"But if my parents ever found out—"

"Don't worry, you'll have the money back tomorrow night. Indian chief's honor."

It meant cutting my first class at school, and inside the

bank I looked around uneasily for adults who might recognize me. But there was no hitch. I took the two tens and a five, folded them tightly and slipped them into Aram's hand before we went back out on the street.

"You're a true brave," he said. "I'll call you as soon as I've got the job."

I squeezed his hand and wished him luck and watched him as he merged into the crowd converging on the subway kiosk. The stairwell swallowed him, and suddenly I knew that I would never see him again.

TO HANDICAPPED TEEN-AGERS: Examine your own feelings and find out whether you are as naive and vulnerable as I was. Aram was an expert; I'm sure that when he looked me over, he tagged me as an easy mark—not just because of my naive manner, but, more important, because of my handicap. I guess he knew he could promise me experiences that I had always believed were out of my reach.

The obvious advice you might expect from me, in light of my encounter with this smooth-talking stranger, would be, "Don't trust a smooth-talking stranger." But looking back on it after all these years, I see it differently.

I have no regrets about being taken in by Aram. When I think of the misery he might have brought to me and my family, I am thankful. I would say that Aram gave me more than he took away.

I am thinking not only of the wooden fan and the amazing little puzzle that he carved for me, but of the lessons that the experience taught me. For one thing, it made me conscious of my need to override the timidity I felt about the way my body looked. I never would have dared to venture into a Greenwich Village hangout looking for "fun," as Aram called it. Certainly the longing was there, but not the courage. This rather drab and sleazy experience left me with a feeling that I could take my new-found wisdom into more beautiful situations.

I don't expect all handicapped teen-agers to have the same feeling I had, but I would like to pass on to them Aram's unintended message—a message of trust. I trusted Aram, and he built on that trust to the point where he got what he wanted ($25)—and then betrayed me.

If you would have that same trust in a similar situation, you could get into really deep trouble because these are different times. If Aram came to your door today, you might immediately wonder whether he might be a burglar, a rapist, or a murderer. But somehow I felt all along that I was protected by my unseen Goddess.

I see this episode as a kind of initiation into a world of reality. If you are as vulnerable as I was, I suggest that you begin testing out some of your fantasies—but without putting yourself in harm's way, as I did. Aram played right into my fantasies—fantasies of being a sophisticated, unafraid, magnetic (to girls) grown-up, as well as a true friend to this interesting stranger. I took my chance on Aram, and I was lucky. I learned to trust, but to trust cautiously. Perhaps you can benefit by my experience.

CHAPTER
13

WHAT ABOUT LOVE?

When I was around nine years old, I became curious about how grown-ups have sex. I recall asking my stepfather to explain this to me; since he was a doctor, I expected him to know all about such matters. But I got no satisfaction. I remember his saying something like, "I'll tell you some other time."

One evening after dinner we were sitting together on a bench in Riverside Park. On the lawn in front of us one little dog was mounting another little dog. Daddy S. pointed them out to me and said, "You wanted to know about sex. There's your answer."

I was puzzled and disappointed. I couldn't believe that this was really my answer. It was just too hard to visualize men and women making love like dogs. But somehow I felt I shouldn't push the matter any further. A year or so later I began finding my own answers—in books.

I took on my own sex education, learning the names of the various parts of the anatomy connected with intercourse, as well as instructions on how to utilize them. I read some of the earlier books, with their dire warnings on masturbation and sex without marriage. Then I read more recent books that contradicted those warnings. I learned about birth control. I filled my head with all kinds of information that really seemed to have nothing to do with the case when I fell in love. But I'm getting ahead of myself.

My first full-blown attraction to a member of the opposite sex came into bloom when I was eleven. Sheila and I met in the Poconos, my family's summer getaway. She had a sweet face and a gentle manner, and she seemed to like walking into the woods with me. We would sit on a fallen tree trunk or a rock and talk about anything. I guess you might call it puppy love—though it had nothing to do with my stepfather's lesson on sex or the little dogs in the park that illustrated it.

Even though there were no letters or phone calls, Sheila stayed in my thoughts all through the following winter and spring. I kept picturing us together, and I wondered why she didn't seem to mind my wearing a brace. In those days boys wore knickerbockers, which covered the legs only down to the knees, so my skinny, braced leg was always conspicuously in view.

When summer came around and it was time to go back to the Poconos, I tensed up with anticipation. Would Sheila be there? Would we still be friends?

She was there, fully as friendly as before. She introduced me to several of her girlfriends, and pretty soon we were all meeting daily for talk and fun. I was the only male member of this group.

One day the game was pin the tail on the donkey. When my turn came, two of the girls blindfolded me and turned me around a few times so I would lose my sense of direction. As I headed straight for the picture of the donkey, I could hear murmurs of admiration. And when I drove the pin into what I thought must be the donkey's backside, there were a few seconds of silence. Then I heard the girls whispering something to the effect of, "Let's move the tail to the donkey's rear end."

As I took the blindfold off, they were all telling me how great I was. I could feel my anger mounting, because I realized instantly that these girls were just trying to give the lame boy a break.

"I heard what you were saying," I told them accusingly. "You moved it!"

There was another moment of silence—an awkward silence this time—and, as nearly as I can remember, the game broke up. After that, Sheila avoided me, or at least I thought she did. Quite possibly I was avoiding her. If there was anything I most emphatically didn't want, it was pity. Even in my adult life I have often felt pity as a form of humiliation.

My "love affair" with Sheila seemed to establish a pattern in my boy-girl relationships: As soon as I sensed that any member of the opposite sex was seriously interested in me, I would turn tail and flee. I couldn't quite believe that an attractive girl would stick with me when she realized my limitations.

Certainly I was not proud of my conduct with Sheila; but looking back I feel even worse about Marie, whom I met four years later. Marie was a waitress in the same establishment. She used no makeup; she let her hair hang straight down, her voice was high-pitched and soft; her manner unassuming and shy. Sometimes she waited on our table, and on these occasions she would linger unnecessarily, fixing her sad eyes on me. Her features were very pretty, but I was not attracted.

Every time our paths crossed, she would give me that same lovelorn look. And when dinner was over, she would seat herself on one of the verandas where she knew I would pass. It got so that when I walked past her I would look straight ahead, as if I didn't know she was there. Many of the guests noticed this; one woman took me aside and said, "You know, Marie is very fond of you, and you make her very unhappy. Why don't you be nice to her?"

I'm afraid her words fell on a stony place inside me. Within that very hour I had to walk past Marie's seat again, and as I did so I got a wrenching sensation. I knew I wasn't being nice. What I didn't know was that I was afraid to give her an advantage over me: If I dared to let her come into my life, she would surely reject me—or so went my thinking.

In any case, I was already in love with Hannah, another waitress there. Her face was lovely and her eyes were a soft gray. The first time she smiled at me, I knew I was in love. For a change, I decided to pursue my desire despite my fears of rejection. She seemed to enjoy walking with me, or sitting on swings side by side, or relaxing on a bench and talking.

I wanted to hug her and kiss her, but I didn't dare to try; I was afraid it would put an end to our enchanted hours together. I kept wondering when I would get up the courage to obey my impulse, but before that question was answered, it was the end of summer and time for us to go home—to different cities.

There were letters—hers newsy, friendly, and noncommittal, mine filled with the passion I couldn't express in person. Hannah did finally agree to a proposal of mine that we spend a day together in Philadelphia, a city equidistant from both our homes. When we met there, I was filled with trepidation, though she was reassuring and friendly.

All through a matinee and dinner, my mouth was sealed. I was even afraid to admit that I wanted to go to the bathroom, lest she feel that I was injecting a note of vulgarity into our date. When at last it was time to part, I said a sheepish good-by and hurried to the men's room.

Several months later I got a letter from Hannah saying that she was soon to be married. I told myself I knew this would happen. It was the old story.

On one of my family's vacations in the Poconos, I became acquainted with a popular girl named Laurie Warner. I was only sixteen or seventeen at the time, but I looked much, much older. Back in Manhattan, Laurie's mother invited me to their apartment for dinner. I had no idea of what to expect. The Warners were longtime friends of my parents, and I thought that perhaps they just wanted to be nice to me. But after dinner they announced that they were going out for the evening and that Laurie would entertain me.

Laurie was a beautiful teen-ager in a pink-and-blond sort of way. I admired her looks and her poise, but so far there was no chemistry between us. Seated on a couch with her, I found myself desperately wondering what to say. Laurie tactfully tried to fill the silences with friendly questions, but she could not relieve my embarrassment.

What kept running through my mind was that neither Laurie nor her parents would ever be willing to allow a handicapped guy like me into their family. But after three or four visits like this, I got, or rather I sensed, the point: They were giving me a chance to woo.

I felt that I mustn't touch this lovely girl, who was so widely admired. Nor must I talk about love or marriage or any kind of intimacy. I must behave. Any deviation from proper behavior, I was sure, would bring swift and crushing rejection.

And behave I did—so much so that even I was bored. I wondered how Laurie could put up with this and why her parents kept inviting me. I became more and more uncomfortable with these visits and finally broke off, still wondering how young men are supposed to comport themselves in the presence of the other sex.

I turned to my brother Ralph for the kind of counseling I

never got from our parents. He must know something, I figured, since he had gone out with quite a few girls. His friendly counseling could not help me overcome the feeling that my handicap made me sexually unattractive, but it didn't stop me from trying.

Ralph and I went to a party at the home of one of his schoolmates, where we were introduced to a petite, vivacious girl who had just moved to New York from Toronto. I was swiftly attracted to her, but was disheartened to see that Ralph was also interested. I was sure I could never compete with him in the boy-meets-girl arena.

Ralph was a slender young man with beautifully sensitive features that made him look like a poet or an artist. He was four years older than I and, I thought, far more sophisticated. Fae was nineteen, compact and sparkly, with pretty features. I was seventeen and lame and ashamed of it.

As the evening wore on, I began to feel that Fae was really interested in me. She accepted Ralph's offer to drive her home, but sat in the back seat of his car with me. She even let me put my arm around her, and before we dropped her at her apartment house, she agreed to a date. I went to bed in a state of euphoria.

This was the beginning of a relationship that went on, with several interruptions, for about four years. During that time we read books together, went to concerts together, partied together, and, when I acquired a canoe, spent long days and weekends together, often picnicking on Hunter Island, one of the little islands that dot Long Island Sound.

On one of our sundown picnics, after the night watchman made his rounds and ordered everybody off the island, we paddled around, watching the sun go down and waiting for the darkness. Then we stealthily glided back to the island and into a little cove we had spotted. We spread a blanket on the ground and bedded down together for the night. It was the first time in my adult life that I had ever lain next to a woman, and my excitement was almost intolerable.

I put an arm around Fae and she snuggled closer to me. But when my free hand started to drift toward forbidden territory, she grabbed my wrist and pulled it away. I tried a few more times, until she said sharply, "Please don't!" Defeated, I spent most of the night in wakeful fantasies about her, alternating with anger at fate for giving me an unattractive body.

Typically, our relationship ended in a quarrel over some trivial incident.

At twenty-one I had never crossed the line into what I considered banned behavior. Helene, who was twenty-three, was the first woman to flash green lights at my wounded ego. One night we were sitting on the grass behind some bushes in Central Park, talking about our writing ambitions and getting as close as we could physically get. Suddenly, to my amazement, Helene unbuttoned her blouse and took off her bra.

We had met at a friend's house just a few days before, but already we were launched on a long, intensely beautiful relationship. Helene would come to my mother's apartment to spend the day collaborating with me on stories or plays and making love. I would visit her at her mother's house to have fun and food with her delightful family. Neither of us were ready, financially or emotionally, to get married, but we relished our very secret love affair. Looking back on it, I think our parents and siblings must have been stone-blind if they did not see what was going on.

Our relationship was smooth and harmonious for two or three years. And then we had a quarrel. I forget what it was about. I was walking Helene from the subway to her home when I said something that offended her. She wanted an apology, but I refused to give her one.

"In that case," Helene said, "I'll never see you again."

I was dumbfounded. I couldn't imagine that my offense was so heinous that she was ready to throw me away. We walked the rest of the way in silence, and at her door we said a cool goodnight.

It was my old pattern coming back after my long, successful battle with it. Of course, I could have called or written or held out some kind of peace offering. But I didn't. Why? Because I was afraid she would reject any advance.

In any case, our affair was an experience I am happy with today. It was more than fun for me; it was emotional growth. Only I still had a long way to go.

———

TO HANDICAPPED LOVERS WITH LOW SELF-ES-TEEM: It is true that some members of the opposite sex won't be interested in you. But many will. Whatever it is that draws one person to another may be based on any of a multitude of factors besides body image—his smile, the way he looks at her, a warmth that communicates itself to her, his facial features, or perhaps the subconscious knowledge that she was attracted to him in a previous lifetime.

I have had patients—male and female—with handicaps far more severe than mine, who have attracted wonderful partners. But admittedly, if you have a highly visible disability, it can make some people feel very uncomfortable for any number of reasons until they get to know you.

People who are interested in more than friendship with you can help you to define your own boundaries and so make the most of your life. That statement calls for some clarification.

Because I am physically disadvantaged, the women who were interested in me were usually well on the road to mental and spiritual growth, and were happy to meet an empathic traveler. These are the beautiful people who helped me stay on that road—or come back to it whenever I strayed. More than that, they are the people who benefited from whatever insights I could offer, thus teaching me that I had something to give to others.

I have counseled many lonely patients, both handicapped and able-bodied, who ask me why it is that they can't find a mate. My answer is always the same: "When you are ready, your mate will be there." My patients rarely believe me, but time after time I get cards and letters from happy ex-patients assuring me that, "Garrett, you were right!"

The bottom line: When you feel that the chemistry is there, have the courage to make your feelings known. Chances are that you will draw a beautiful response.

———

TO THE BELOVED OF A HANDICAPPED PERSON: What will your friends think? If you love a handicapped young man or woman, don't let that question bother you. Most of them will admire you for it. But if any of them get the idea that he's "the best she could get," educate them! Show them by your own example that a handicap need never interfere with true love and that happiness is not dependent on the way people look.

If you truly love a handicapped person, you will get a deep satisfaction out of understanding his special needs. This in turn can help you to understand that every individual has special needs—that the world is not divided into the lame and the able-bodied, the rich and the poor, the strong and the weak, or any other pair of opposites. It can help you to realize that every person occupies a special place in the human spectrum.

CHAPTER
14

THE MAGICAL WORLD
OF DADDY O.

As my interests shifted more and more toward the kind of life that might be open to me, like writing and the arts, I'm afraid I developed a self-serving sense of superiority toward the robust physicality of Daddy S. When Daddy O. and Mother O. and my brother Ralph moved back from California, I began skipping my homework and taking the bus to Washington Square every night to spend an hour or two with them.

Somewhere around this time (I was about fourteen) I took this visionary poet and parent as my role model. And I began badgering my trio of parents for permission to live with him. As usual, I was able to get my way.

Daddy O. lived with my new stepmother, whom I looked on as more of a wonderful companion than a parent, and my brother Ralph. They were settled in a picturesque rooming house on the south side of Washington Square. It was run by an elderly French landlady named Madame Blanchard, or simply Madame. From Daddy O.'s third-floor window, you could see over the famous Washington Arch straight up Fifth Avenue. Ralph occupied a smaller room, where he wrote blood-and-thunder stories. My school was a long subway ride away.

Now Ralph and I moved into the large rear room that connected with my father's by a corridor that was fixed up as a bathroom. We spent many evenings in the front room, where I would listen with rapt attention while Daddy O. would interpret my brother's long and fascinating dreams.

Daddy O. had studied with the great Carl Jung in Switzerland and had practiced for many years as a Jungian therapist. But at this time he was devoting his energies to writing.

Sitting, almost literally, at his feet, I gently absorbed some of the major Jungian concepts—the collective unconscious, the psychological types, the meaning of dreams, the eternal feminine. All these ideas meshed somehow with my own spiritual experiences. A whole new magical world was opening up to me.

Moreover, Daddy O. had some wonderful visitors—artists, novelists, poets, composers, even a well-known cartoonist. This world was the magic carpet on which I, the Little Lame Prince, could ride to a more tangible contact with the universe—one that I might even be able to articulate. It was a kind of grown-up version of my favorite fairy tale.

More and more I yearned to get out of high school and live a life of the spirit.

One of the most wonderful attractions of my new life style was Mother O., who had immediately befriended and captivated me. She was a very delicate-looking woman who loved flowery dresses and big hats. She had a soft voice and she painted exquisite pictures, which were all around the room she shared with my father.

I was particularly charmed by the story of Mother O.'s daring invasion of Washington Arch. She had discovered a door in the arch that was left unlocked. Going through the door, she found a stairway that took her to the top.

In the dead of night, Mother O. and a group of her artist friends, including John Sloan and Marcel Duchamp, climbed to the top, where they had a party to celebrate the secession of Greenwich Village from the United States. Next morning this historic landmark was festooned with colorful gas balloons. A highly amusing and somewhat different version of this story appeared in the May 13, 1991, issue of the *New Yorker* magazine.

Mother O. and I would take long walks together, and our friendship developed an almost conspiratorial air. On one of these walks a gray-bearded man with glasses came to her side and moved into step with us. He began talking in a low voice.

I couldn't make out what he was saying, but I could see that Mother O. wanted him to leave us alone. At first I wondered why she didn't tell him to go away, but then I gathered that she was afraid of him. Her fear communicated itself to me. I found myself wishing that I was able-bodied and strong enough to demolish this man. He didn't leave us until we reached the stoop of our home.

One night as we were all talking in the front room, this man appeared in the open doorway without saying a word. Daddy O., who was much smaller than the intruder, sprang from his chair and pushed him out into the hallway. Without speaking, he jostled him all the way to the top of the stairs and with a final push sent him tumbling down.

Fred Lewis, as I soon learned was his name, picked himself up, found his glasses on the floor, and shouted drunkenly, "Oppenheim, I'm going to come up there and cut your bowels out!"

I was frozen in my chair until my father came back, breathing hard and looking extremely angry. This was the only time I ever saw him fighting or looking that way. I gathered that Fred Lewis had done him some terrible wrong, but I couldn't imagine what it was. Looking back, I can only guess that this unhappy drunkard was trying to force his attentions on my stepmother. My father was a gentle, peace-loving man—anything but a fighter. He must have been severely angered to attack Fred Lewis in this manner.

It was an unpleasant lesson for me—a lesson that every child who watches television these days has learned only too well: the almost unacceptable truth that some men try to force their attentions on unwilling women.

Every once in a while, after that, we could hear Fred Lewis out on the street, shouting his obscene threats to my father. I never found out whatever happened to this sick individual, but presently he seemed to dissolve from the scene—in a lake of alcohol, I would guess.

I had been writing poetry since the age of eleven, but now I was pouring it out, hoping for accolades from my father. Looking back, I blush at the overall poor quality of my efforts. My father read them dutifully, pointing out errors in grammar and spelling, and giving me his expert evaluations. He never told me what to write or how; he was simply helpful and supportive.

Presently some of my poems were accepted for publication in prestigious papers and magazines. And one night, talking about Ralph's successes and mine, Daddy O. made this remark: "It's as if my two sons were carrying out two unfulfilled interests of mine—to write popular fiction and popular poetry."

The significance of the word "popular" wasn't lost on me. I knew that he meant "shallow," in contrast to "deep," which was the way he—and I—rated his own work. Once more he seemed to be telling me that despite his love he saw me largely as a less important part of himself—a part he had not seen fit to cultivate.

The magic world that he had opened up for me seemed to recede beyond my reach. My poems were just the expression of a very unfulfilled but secondary part of Daddy O. After a year of living with him, I could feel, without ever admitting it to my consciousness, that he did not see me or accept me as a person in my own right. It was the same message I got on my tenth birthday, when I read his reaction to the discovery that I had polio.

Mother O. told me my poems were wonderful. Talking with her always made me feel good about myself. Just as Ralph and I divided all people into trolls and nontrolls, she called people lemons and poppies. She published a book of line drawings depicting both types, and the correspondence of lemons to trolls was remarkable.

My favorite lemon was the portrait of a lean, long-jawed woman who was President of the Society for the Prevention of Watching Isadora Duncan Dance. That revolutionary dancer had shocked the nation's gatekeepers of morality by baring her breasts during a performance.

One day Mother O. divulged a secret: She and her friend Nadia Sanzewich had rented a store at the west edge of Greenwich Village, where they planned to feature my book, *Lyrics to the Olympian Deities*, which I had written at the age of twelve. Moreover, they were going to put copies of the book in the window. And she showed me some beautiful jackets she had painted to go over the drab cardboard covers of the book.

Nadia and Mother O. and I all went together to the store to begin fixing it up. The store was down a few steps, because, as our vivacious Nadia put it, "People like better to go down than up." Nadia, Mother O. confided in me, was a Russian princess who had come to our country incognito to escape the Czar's wrath.

A Russian princess! Wow! I don't think I will ever know whether this was true or a concoction of Mother O.'s energetic imagination. But to me it was just more magic.

I was exhilarated by the sight of the jacketed copies of my book in the window; you could see them from the street. As you may have guessed, there were no sales, and somehow the store project dissolved. Moreover, I was asked to keep it all a secret, even from Daddy O.

In spite of the project's collapse, the experience stands out in my memory as a very happy one—no doubt, because Mother O. was showing me the kind of care and support I never quite got from Daddy O.

I loved my father. I respected him. I'm sure I must have exchanged hugs with this wonderful man many times; but strangely enough, I have no memory of those hugs.

I do have a memory of an argument between Daddy and Mother O. that opened my eyes to a universal problem: misunderstanding.

Our little family generally had dinner at Joe's Italian restaurant on Bleecker Street. Mother O. had been to her dentist that afternoon; she reported that he had advised her to brush her teeth back and forth, rather than up and down. Daddy O. gently reminded her that some six months ago this same dentist had advised brushing the teeth up and down—never sideways.

Mother O: Well, they keep on doing research, and this is what they're now saying.

Daddy O: How can you put stock in anything they tell you when they keep changing their minds?

M: Well, they can only give you the best up-to-date information, don't you agree?

D: You're missing my point. If they keep changing what they say, how can you believe them?

M: You just take the latest as the best they can give you.

D: You're missing my point. . . .

It went on like that until Daddy O. was getting exasperated and tears were welling up in Mother O.'s eyes. I wanted to intervene and say, "Both of you are right. Can't you see that?" But I was too shy to step in between these two idols. The tension hovered over us all through dinner.

I don't know whether this amazing quarrel over trivia was an indication of a much deeper rift that was developing between these two wonderful people. At the time I remained silent, but I kept turning over this argument in my mind until I came up with the obvious conclusion: There is never just one way of looking at something.

Is this the reason why people fight wars? Is this why couples get divorced? Is this why Mother O. mysteriously faded out of our lives? I never found out the answer to that last question, and for some reason I could never bring myself to ask Daddy O. about it, but it left me with a sadness and an emptiness.

Some time later, Daddy O. introduced me to a woman named Linda, who lived in the same building. She was a shy, soft-spoken young English woman who was soon part of our evening *mise en scéne*. A few months later Linda became my father's third wife.

TO PARENTS, STEPPARENTS, AND SURROGATES: When a family constellation is crisscrossed by divorce and remarriage, there are bound to be many crisis times. While the teen years may be difficult for almost any youngster, they can sometimes put mountains in the path of the handicapped one, whose fears of abandonment often connect directly with his body image.

If in addition his biological parents are divorced and one or both are remarried, and they are all on the scene, the stage is set for a web of psychological troubles.

When you sense that something's not right with your handicapped son or daughter, a good way to get him to open up is to do things with him. Go fishing or golfing, camp out for a weekend, take long auto trips to interesting places. And when you and he are doing these things together, there will be many opportunities to talk.

You can obliquely bring up the subject of his feelings. For example, "What kind of man do you most admire?" Or gently and directly—as, "You don't seem to be your old self lately. Something bugging you?"

Never ask yourself—or anybody else—"What did I do wrong?" But rather, "How can I help?" Remember that touching has extraordinary healing powers. Hugging or kissing a handicapped youngster or simply putting an arm around his shoulders sends him a clear communication that you are not put off by his limp or the way his body looks. It can also build in him a message of hope—hope that someday some desirable person of the opposite sex will find him attractive.

If, as in my case, he has three or four parents, any serious quarreling between any of them can reanimate his old conflict of loyalties and his fear of abandonment by one or more of them.

A teen-ager should be convinced that he is no longer a helpless child, such as I was in my earliest dream, where I was unable to choose a daddy; by now he is eligible to make choices. If he does make a choice and acts on it, he may presently find himself in trouble, wondering if he can ever restore things to the way they were.

Divorced parents and stepparents would do well to alert themselves to the first signs of this problem and take measures before it becomes acute.

What are the signs? Suppose you are the mother or step-father, living together with your son. You note that he is spending more time with his biological father than with you. He is losing interest in school and getting poorer grades. He is thinking of going into the same kind of career as his absent father. He tends to be moody and morose. He disagrees with almost anything you say. He picks quarrels with you. If a stepbrother has been added to the family, he accuses you of playing favorites. Finally he announces that he wants to live with his "real" father.

At this point, putting your foot down on his demand would only add to the antagonisms. Tell him, instead, that it might be a good idea to further his development. But at the same time be sure to let him know that your door is open any time he wants to come back.

CHAPTER
15

DEATH OF A MYSTIC WARRIOR

"Death—as commonly spoken of—is only passing through God's other door." Edgar Cayce reading 1472-2

During our many summer discussions of life and death on the steps in front of Madame's rooming house, Daddy O. came up with this request: "Please don't put me into a cemetery when I go. I would like my body to be cremated and the ashes sprinkled on Madame's stoop on a slippery day." I wasn't sure whether or not he was joking. I finally had to assume he was.

Daddy O. died at the age of fifty from a constellation of illnesses brought on largely by poverty and Prohibition liquor. I was too young and green to take charge, and his third wife, Linda, was too shaken up, as was my brother Ralph.

My father's brothers arranged for a large funeral service at which Dr. John Lovejoy Elliot, president of the Ethical

Culture Society, delivered an eloquent eulogy. He had been a good friend of my father's in the days when Daddy O. was active in social reform projects, but the two friends had not seen or heard from each other in at least two decades.

I listened with emotion to Dr. Elliot's description of the young James Oppenheim as a spiritual visionary, dedicated to social causes for the poor. In the middle of this, Linda, who was sitting next to me in the front row, interrupted, saying, "That's not the way James was!"

There was a moment of dead silence. I reached for Linda's arm and gave it a squeeze to forestall a possible debate. Then Dr. Elliot picked up on the situation and said gently, "I am talking about the James Oppenheim I knew." And he went right on with his eulogy.

When the service was over, I, the easily embarrassed one, left the auditorium in a state of grief mixed with depression and confusion.

We got into the lead car, and I was conscious of our funeral procession winding its way through the city and out to Long Island. "The snake of death," I said to myself mentally.

At the crematory, we gathered in a small auditorium. My Uncle Robert came over and asked me if I would like to say a few words. "I can't," I said lamely, hoping he would understand my grief.

There was another reason why I declined: I just didn't want to limp up to the platform. In some way, I felt, the sympathy for my disability would detract from the grief we all felt at our loss. As for Ralph, he was obviously too shaken up even to be asked. So Uncle Robert gave a short ad lib farewell talk about his brother.

After that, Ralph and I watched in a kind of mental paralysis as the casket was wheeled to position in front of a special door. As it was slowly pushed through, I knew in my gut that this was the last of my father's body. I couldn't help wondering whether this was the right thing to do. I had read about the Egyptians, who preserved the body of the deceased so that the spirit could return into it. I knew intellectually that I'd rather see a body turned to ashes than have it eaten by worms. Ralph and I both felt an awesome finality as the elevator went down to the furnace.

Weeks later, when I went back to the crematory to pick up the ashes, all that remained of my father's earthly reality was given to me in a container about the size of a coffee can. Ralph and Linda were happy to let me take charge of them. I took the container home and kept it in my room through the winter months, communicating frequently with my father's beautiful spirit. I could not bring myself to perform the indignity my father had jokingly requested. So when spring came, I took the can to City Island and rented a rowboat.

I rowed farther and farther out until I had a feeling of undisturbed solitude. Then I pulled in the oars and picked up the container. After holding it for several minutes, I took the cover off and took a long last look at what once had the semblance of my father.

"Good-by, Dad," I whispered, and shook the ashes out into the calm waters.

A growing certainty came to me: This was not the last of my father. This was not the end of our love. The image of my beloved Goddess seemed to rise out of the water.

TO PARENTS AND OTHER CONCERNED ADULTS: When a child of any age asks questions, truthful responses from a person he loves and respects are a great strengthener. This is particularly pertinent when the child wants to know about death. Avoiding a discussion of this most feared and most inevitable event can only make it seem more terrible.

Every child wants to know, of course, whether he will go on existing after he dies. The handicapped child may also want some additional information. If you have told him of your own belief that he will go on, he may ask, "When I die, will I still be lame (or blind, or deaf, or whatever)?"

Just telling him not to worry, that everything will be all right, is ducking the issue and probably sending him the message that (a) death is too awful to be talked about and (b) he'll still have his handicap.

There are many belief systems about death, and you probably have some beliefs of your own. I would say, show respect for your child's desire to learn and answer as truthfully as you can within the framework of your own beliefs.

Children generally do not ask about such things as sex and death until they are ready to hear the answers. Your response can, of course, be framed in gentle, reassuring words. If you truly believe that bodily death is the end of the soul's existence, I would advise against inventing fairy tales about Heaven. Children have a fine-tuned ear that usually tells them when they are being taken.

My own conviction, based on many years as a past-life therapist, is that we reincarnate—that we have lived before and will come back to live again. I would express this to a child as my belief, but not something I can really know for sure.

If my questioner is old enough to understand, I would explain the concept of karma, the idea that we are constantly evolving from life to life, and that the problems we don't face up to in one life will be given to us again in another, and another, until we deal with them. The laws of karma also tell us that if we have done wrong in a past life, we will suffer wrong in a subsequent life so that we can learn what it feels like to be at the other end of the stick.

Thus you can explain to the handicapped child that his

disability was given to him so that he might learn from it, and perhaps pass that learning on to others. If he takes advantage of his opportunities in this life, there will be no need for him to be handicapped in the next one.

The prospect of reincarnating with an able body can help to make death seem like a big step in that direction and take much of the fear out of it. It can also motivate the child to learn everything he can, even when he grows old enough to know that death is near. The more learning he has assimilated in this life, the wiser he will be in the next.

That is the way I would speak to a child today, based on my own experiences and all the scientific evidence for reincarnation that I have read and heard about. You, good reader, may have entirely different ideas, and I would urge you to explain death and handicaps to your young questioner in accordance with your beliefs.

If you believe in some kind of heaven in the hereafter, you might explain that you see death as just the doorway to a wonderful new kind of life—life without any handicap—and that now is the time for him to prepare for that life by ridding himself of anger and hate and all the other destructive emotions.

But suppose you don't believe in any kind of afterlife, but you are firmly convinced that death is the end of existence—that "dust thou art, to dust returnest" applies to the soul as well as the body. Then your job is going to be harder. Telling a child that death means annihilation is an almost certain way of implanting terror in his heart and bringing on nightmares. The handicapped child in particular may feel cheated out of his only chance for a life with a sound body and mind. To avoid this, I would suggest that you say something along the following lines:

"Nobody really knows what happens to us after death, but for many thousands of years people have seen it as a happy existence. I have often thought about it, but I can't say that I know more than anybody else. Every person must get his own feelings about it. If you just think about it now and then, perhaps some answer will come to you. But in the meantime you can be thankful for the beautiful gift of life that you now have."

The important point to remember is that children are just as scared of death as many adults nearing the end of life. So this is an area in which good parenting is vital—especially if your young questioner is handicapped.

CHAPTER
16

FAREWELL TO STRONG
AND LOVING ARMS

We all knew that Daddy S. had a heart condition. But at the age of fifty-four he was getting around energetically. He had a springy step and a dynamic manner that inspired confidence in his patients and in his family. None of us took the diagnosis too seriously, since there was no visible sign of danger. He himself didn't seem to be bothered by it; he was making his rounds and caring for his heavy load of patients as usual, even making house calls that were far out of his way.

At the time I'm speaking of—my twentieth year, that is—we had a live-in maid named Tessie—a tall, rosy-cheeked, stereotypical picture of a European peasant—honest, cheerful, and endlessly energetic. Tessie spent her weekends with her husband, John, and her eleven-year-old son. They lived on the fifth floor of a walk-up on the lower East Side.

One Monday, when our parents were already out for the day, Tessie came to work in tears. Her husband, she told us, was near death, and she didn't know any way to get medical help for him. In those days there was no 9-1-1.

I took charge of the situation, as I was in the habit of doing, and told Tessie not to worry. "I'll speak to my Dad," I said. "He'll make an emergency call on John tonight."

At the dinner table later on, Daddy S. looked tired, but I felt that this was a life-and-death matter. I told him about Tessie's husband and her total inability to pay a doctor. I said, "I told Tessie you would never turn your back on a dying man."

Daddy S. frowned. To my surprise, he said he was almost too tired to climb four flights of stairs after a full day's work.

Seeing his hesitation, I asked, "What are you going to do?" I was unaware of the seriousness of his heart condition.

Shortly after dinner Daddy S. left the house to save John's life if he could. It was several hours later before he returned, in a state of extreme exhaustion—and anger.

"It was just a bad cold," he said. "John'll be better by morning. He didn't need a doctor."

He changed into his nightclothes and flopped into a steamer chair which he had set up in the living room to slow his heart. I could see him taking his own pulse from time to time.

Three days later there was a crisis. My mother and I hurried to Daddy S.'s side. He was in the steamer chair, hyperventilating; he talked to us with great difficulty. "I'm sick," he said. We stayed at his side, bringing him whatever help he asked for. His breathing calmed down somewhat, and one by one we got ready for sleep.

But about 2:30 in the morning his breathing sounded worse than ever, and we went back to his chair. He told me to go to Wasself's Pharmacy, which was three or four blocks away, and ask for a bottle of nitroglycerine. "Tell Mr. Wasself

I'll send the prescription along tomorrow," he added.

Within minutes I was racing through the streets as fast as my brace and cane would take me. Fifteen minutes later I was back with the life-saving drug. Daddy S., still in charge of his own case, told me how to administer it to him. After he got the medication under his tongue, he settled back in the steamer chair, still breathing heavily, but not so alarmingly. As time went by, his breathing subsided into a steady, loud rhythm.

Mom and I finally felt we could retire, but the sound of Daddy S.'s breathing followed us into our sleep. Suddenly we heard a gasp, and then there was complete silence. We both knew immediately what it meant. I hurried to get into my brace and clothes and joined my mother at chairside. I picked up Daddy S.'s arm to feel his pulse, but the arm was already cold.

Along with my alarm, I could feel the guilt racing through my veins. If I had not insisted that Daddy S. make that useless house call, maybe he would still be alive. Did I, in effect, murder him?

I did not express this horrible thought—not even to my brother Ralph. I just allowed it to build up inside of me.

My mother immediately called her brother Walter, who was also a physician, and a half-hour later he was in our apartment taking charge. Uncle Walter was a man with a sadistic sense of humor, a man I had come to fear as a child. On his frequent visits to our home, he would amuse himself by squeezing me between his knees and tickling me vigorously. When I screamed for him to stop, he would squeeze and tickle harder. On one visit, when I was about twelve, he returned my welcome by spitting all over my face. My reaction, of course, was to wonder what made me bad enough to justify such a display of contempt.

Uncle Walter summoned an ambulance and then called on the night elevator operator to help him. At his direction, the elevator man took the feet while Uncle Walter grabbed Daddy S. under the armpits. When they lifted the body, Daddy S.'s head jerked backward and hung loosely, swaying and bouncing while they carried him out.

The sight filled me with anger, and then with an awesome sense of the finality of death. This exuberant man, who had cared for me and radiated love for his family, was being carried away like so much garbage. Only later did I begin to understand that this was not the man; it was a housing. But I never forgave Uncle Walter for his callousness in the midst of our bereaved family.

Incidentally, my brother Louis remained in his bedroom all through this drama. I believe it was too much for him to witness.

———

TO THE HANDICAPPED: As you've seen throughout this book, my disability always seemed to be an aggravating factor, if not the cause, of self-damaging thoughts. The death of a parent can trigger extreme feelings of guilt. The handicapped person, already an expert at finding reasons to blame himself, consciously or unconsciously, will immediately ask himself, "What did I do to bring this about?"

In my case, the question was easy to answer: I had nagged my stepfather into a useless midnight trip involving four flights of stairs to treat a man who didn't need a doctor. This was aggravated by the growing realization that, much as I idolized Daddy O., Daddy S. had always been my real father—the father who was there for me. Memories flooded me—memories of all the doctoring, all the outings, all the games, all the evidences of love he had showered on me all through my childhood.

It took me some years and a lot of professional help to

cope with all these feelings, which I tried to deny. I am writing this down in the hope that I may spare others the kind of self-laceration I carried inside me.

What can you do when you must face up to the death of a parent? First of all, realize that your conduct was not so much a matter of choice as a matter of circumstance. Perhaps the most important factor is your handicap, which any child could interpret as a punishment for being bad. In my case, my Daddy O.'s view—that I was a symbol of his wrecked marriage—had already ratcheted these feelings to a dangerously high level.

I think I finally released myself from my own guilt and shame about my relations with Daddy S. With professional help I was able to admit to myself that my attitude was unfortunate, but also to understand how experiences beyond my immature control had governed me.

I imagine that many handicapped individuals, if they search, can come up with similar traumatizing experiences. So I would say to anyone with a history much like mine, look both outward and inward. Examine the causes of your bad feelings about yourself. Analyze the ways the outward circumstances played on your vulnerabilities, and then release yourself from the terrible weight of guilt you carry within you.

CHAPTER
17

THE GREAT DEPRESSION—
AND MINE

My father's exciting revelations about the unconscious had spurred me on into a deeper and deeper search of my own inner world. I began writing down my dreams and analyzing them the way Daddy O. had taught me. I knew about the meaning of free association and of the link between inspired poetry and analytic psychology. I began reading the books my father admired. But I was living what the world called an unproductive life. Part of me had to agree with that verdict.

Daddy O. and Daddy S. had died within a year of each other, leaving me at loose ends, psychologically. My dreams and fantasies would not let me relinquish my search for a spiritual meaning to my life. I went to poetry meetings and attended classes with such poets as W. H. Auden, Kenneth Fearing, and other searchers. I longed to get into psychoanalysis, because I believed that it would help me find the answers for which I had been seeking for so many years. But I was low on funds.

At around this time, however, I learned about Lewis Wolberg, a prominent New York psychiatrist who was also doing some pioneering work in hypnosis. He had founded a clinic for people who couldn't pay the usual fees. The clinic's charge was eight dollars for a fifty-minute session.

I had a few exploratory sessions with him, involving some probing interviews and a Rorschach test, in which you look at some blobby ink-blot shapes and report what you see in them. Then I was assigned to a very capable young psychiatrist who belonged to what was known as the Washington School—a group that followed Freudian concepts, but with significant modification. I worked intensively with him and then with two other young psychiatrists of the same school for a total of eleven years.

Results? Some very valuable help on immediate problems, but no great revelations. I finally quit with a feeling of disap-pointment. Nevertheless, these sessions proved to be excel-lent training for the profession I was to enter many years later.

I remember talking freely to my analysts about my family relationships, about my social inhibitions, about my shaky self-esteem. But rarely—very rarely—did we get around to the subject of my handicap and how it had affected my life.

I still remember telling my first analyst why it was so impossible for me to get a job and make a living. I cited my inexperience, the Great Depression, my lack of a college diploma, etc., etc. I remember how his eyes narrowed as they seemed to bore into my psyche, and how he impressed me with a memorable remark that I now use with some of my own patients.

"The stable stinks," he said, "but it's warm."

I was soon prodded into action. The Great Depression had demoralized the whole country, and I was pretty much demoralized myself. The kind of jobs I wanted were impossible to get without a college diploma. Daddy O., my role model, never went through college; yet he was held in great esteem by many writers, artists, and educators. I figured I didn't need a sheepskin either. But times were changing.

I had quit high school in my junior year to go to music school, and then quit music school to look for a job, and then quit looking because there just were no jobs. So my prospects at this point were decidedly poor.

But I had to get out of that stable!

With the help of friends, I sent out about fifty hand-typed letters offering my services as a writer or editor. Two or three of my letters drew replies turning me down. The rest were ignored.

Trudging along the streets of Manhattan, I passed any number of lines for soup kitchens. I passed signs on Sixth Avenue that also drew long lines; the signs said, "Wanted—Dishwasher—$8 a week" (a week, not a day!). The papers carried so many stories of executives jumping out of windows in the Wall Street area that it got to be routine reading. And there just were no jobs.

But was it really the Depression that kept me in idleness, I wondered, or was it me? The kind of job I wanted, I was told everywhere, called for a college diploma—and I was a high-school dropout. The kind of job I would have settled for—loading trucks or delivering flowers—called for an able body—and again, I was disqualified.

I was living at home with my widowed mother and my younger brother Lou, who was at school. Aside from job-hunting, I spent my time practicing piano, talking with friends, reading, and writing poetry, which I got to be quite good at. Though much of my poetry was accepted by respectable publications and won kudos from fellow poets, there was no real money in it. In my best year my poems earned me $100.05.

My older brother Ralph was earning a living with his short stories. Lou was studying for his bachelor's degree at Columbia University. My mother was working very hard as a public-school teacher to keep us going. But I was contributing nothing to my family, and I felt terribly ashamed about it. Though my feelings and my analysis impelled me to step up my job search, that was the most unproductive task of all.

About this time I made the acquaintance of Florence Hamilton, a matronly poet who lived across the street just a couple of hundred feet from my home. Florence was intensely interested in parapsychological phenomena, which she had been studying for many years.

I became a constant guest at her home, which was jam-packed with books. They occupied an entire wall of the long hallway in her apartment and crowded many of the rooms. I enjoyed long talks with Florence, and though I didn't think too much of her poetry, I could not help admiring this literary lady.

When Florence learned that I was interested in metaphysics, she showed me some of her many historical books on spiritualism and psychic phenomena. In particular she let me have, on a long-term loan, a remarkable book by Baron Von Schrenck Notzing, translated from the German. Von Schrenck Notzing, a psychiatrist with a good scientific background, had performed many experiments to authenticate or disprove the existence of spirits.

The thick book detailed some of his experiments with well-known mediums. To make sure that there was no possibility of fraud, he would strip and search his volunteer and seat her on a hard chair. The book was illustrated with amazing photographs, taken with flash sheets. They showed clouds of ectoplasm emanating from the medium's naked body.

It is hard to believe that a man of Von Schrenck Notzing's

reputation and acknowledged integrity would fake such pictures. I believed in them, particularly as I had myself seen entities from realms beyond our knowledge. The book haunts me, but I have never been able to unearth a copy of it. Recently, however, a good friend found a companion volume for me by the same author. It's titled *Phenomena of Materialisation* and features an even greater abundance of convincing photographs. This reprint was published by Arno Press in 1975.

Florence had a niece named Thelma, who became a close friend of mine for many years. She and I spent many hours of my unemployment time, reading books together and speculating on the world beyond the world we know.

Meanwhile, the whole country was beginning to be occupied with the threat of war. The *New York Times* reports pushed other interests aside with their harrowing descriptions of the Holocaust. I listened in disbelief and horror to the hate messages Hitler would spew out on the radio. It gave me the feeling that my own little troubles were nothing in the face of the wholesale annihilation of human beings.

Then came the beginning of World War II in Europe, and our own country, galvanized, began girding for battle. Everywhere the draft was taking our able-bodied young men away from their homes and their jobs. I had a burning desire to do something, anything I could, to fight this incredible savagery.

I was called up before the draft board and promptly rejected. Thelma's husband, Al, was called up around the same time and promptly accepted.

I still wanted to be part of the war effort, and I soon found my own way. Along with Thelma, I volunteered to serve as an air warden. These unsung non-heroes and -heroines had the thankless job of getting people off the streets and into safety whenever the air-raid sirens sounded. Since shooting at real human beings was utterly repellent to me, I was delighted to have a task that might save lives instead of destroying them. I was also delighted with the whole new circle of friends I acquired in this service.

After some training and a little practice on the streets of my neighborhood, I became Deputy Sector Commander of our unit. The commander (my superior) ran a business that took the greater part of his time; so in effect I was making most of the decisions for our unit.

In one way this jacked up my fragile ego; in another way I felt it as a downer. It played on my deeper feeling that I was in this position because (a) I was unfit to serve in the armed forces and (b) I was unemployed. To nourish my ego, I intensified my search for a job.

My brother Lou graduated from college and presently moved to Pittsburgh, where he become a respected executive in the echelons of Westinghouse. Ralph was still writing stories for a popular magazine. I was rattling around from long periods of unemployment to odd—yes, very odd— jobs. I wrote poems, I listened to music, I had long talks with friends, and particularly with Ralph, on jobs, politics, women, the world—and I nursed my own depression in private. My mother kept impressing on me, sometimes lovingly, sometimes angrily, that I wasn't fit to hold a job.

A friend told me about the great Saturday afternoon organ concerts at the Cathedral of Saint John the Divine, which was just a short walk from my home. I soon got the habit of making this a regular weekly occasion. It gave me a chance to communicate with the great Creative Power, which I felt I was in danger of losing.

The stained-glass windows of the cathedral filtered the sunlight through colors that seemed to bring messages from another realm—messages of comfort and assurance. They were inspiring in themselves. These brief interludes were probably the steadiest spiritual refreshment I had in those days. I would come home feeling renewed and ready to take on another week of whatever my destiny offered.

It brought me an offer of sorts. The wife of a German orchestra conductor was writing children's operettas and needed an English-speaking lyricist/librettist. I was referred to her by a friend of my mother's. The freelance job paid meagerly, but I was treated to fine lunches in my employer's brownstone house on the upper East Side. I also had the pleasure of talking music with her husband, who had retired as conductor of the Berlin Philharmonic orchestra. I told him how much I admired Toscanini, and I remember how he shook his head disapprovingly.

"Too fast, too fast," he said. "Like a machine."

While I was working on the operettas, ASCAP (American Society of Composers and Publishers), the powerful union representing the songwriters, went on strike. The union successfully banned all radio stations from broadcasting songs by its members.

A friend who knew I could write lyrics referred me to a music publishing house named Langlois and Wentworth, where I was interviewed by Cy Langlois, the chief executive. Without further ado, he showed me into a beautiful, spacious office with windows overlooking Madison Avenue. I did not realize at the time that I was sort of a strikebreaker. I was paid $15 a week.

My job was to take the music by some composers who worked for the same firm and put lyrics to them. Sometimes I even created both words and music. I was able to put the melody down on paper, but nothing more. However, when I hummed my tune, with one of the composers seated at a piano, he would come up with a nice arrangement for it. Sometimes I had the thrill of turning on the radio and hearing one of my creations.

I signed my name Gene Stark, because I felt the songs did not represent the kind of spiritual person I felt I was. But every once in a while I would try to create something more in character. My favorite lyric, which I set to my own music, went like this:

Verse:
>   Once upon a time, in the land of Eden,
>   Lived a man of clay.
>   He didn't know writin', he didn't know readin',
>   But he sure knew how to pray!

Chorus:
>   Adam in a garden stood,
>   Shoutin' loud, as loud as he could,
>   "O Lawd, I'm lonely!
>   Won'tcha gimme someone to love?"
>
>   And the Lawd, he heard that prayer.
>   He responded out o' the air,
>   "If you is lonely,
>   Gonna give you someone to love."
>
>   So he fetched a bride
>   Out of Adam's side
>   While Adam lay a-sleepin'.
>   Then Adam woke,
>   And up he spoke:
>   "O Lawd, is findin's keepin'?"
>
>   That's the way it all began.
>   Ever since that original man,
>   We all get lonely
>   When there ain't someone to love.

While I enjoyed this kind of work, I did not discontinue my long search for a more secure job. My efforts finally paid off. I wangled an interview with Bill Kirby, the editor of the *Wall Street Journal.* This friendly man told me that with the shortage of manpower in the business world, his paper was relaxing its requirement of a college diploma. Though he had no editorial job opening at the moment, he invited me to keep in touch.

That same day I went to the circulation department and was given a clerical job, which I held for several weeks. Not a very inspiring situation, but for me it was a stepping-stone to the editorial staff.

Every working day I paid a visit to Bill Kirby. And every day he told me, "Not yet." But the day came when he surprised me with, "I'll try you out." And the next thing I knew, I was on the copy desk, earning a living.

The copy desk, at least as I knew it, is at the heart of the newspaper's operation. It is usually built in a U-shape, and the copy editors sit around the rim of it. They are known as "rim men" (even though there are women on the desk). The chief of the desk sits in the inside, or "slot," of the circle.

Every story handed in by the reporters and feature writers is funneled through the slot man, who decides what kind of headline to put on it and passes it on to one of the rim men. The rim man reads the story carefully for sense, appropriate position of paragraphs, language, typographical correctness, and so forth, then writes a headline on it. Headlines must conform to rigid style rules, and each line must exactly fit the allotted space.

Though I had done my homework, I was somewhat overwhelmed by the demands this job made for judgment and precision. But I was also fired up by the giant step I had taken from guilt-ridden unemployment to glorious independence. No one, I think, was more surprised than my mother. I was finally in a class with my two brothers. I no longer felt so apologetic for being alive. In fact I was just beginning to accept myself.

The camaraderie of the little group on the copy desk was good medicine for me. My feelings of isolation dissolved a little more every day. Our workday started at four in the afternoon, so every evening we all went together to our choice of the local restaurants. Going to and from our dinner, there was never any sign of impatience with my slower gait.

But now another problem developed: The head of the copy desk, a man with a temper as sharp as his mind, seemed to resent my presence on his team—maybe because I was the only copy editor without a college diploma, or maybe because in some way my disability riled him. Goldie, as we called him, picked on me so regularly and so conspicuously that one night, as I learned later, the other copy editors took him aside and suggested that he cut it out. He toned his attacks down, and within a few weeks after that we were very good friends.

A few of us, including Goldie, took the same subway line home every night. Since the trains ran less frequently at this late hour, Goldie was always in a hurry to make a certain express that would save him ten minutes or so. I felt his haste as a pressure on me to walk faster than I should.

In those days I was able to walk at a fairly good clip, but I was at some risk when I tried to keep up with Goldie. Stepping off a curb one night, I put my cane down on a manhole cover. It went right into one of the little holes in the cover, taking me with it as it plunged down. The crook on top of the cane saved it from disappearing, but didn't stop me from having a nasty spill.

What hurt me most was not the painful shock to my body, but an immediate and horrible feeling that I was making a ludicrous spectacle of myself. When I got back on my feet, I actually felt that I should apologize to my friends. It was the old concern with the way I must look to others. Would I ever live it down?

TO HANDICAPPED PEOPLE WITH LOW SELF-ES-TEEM: When your self-esteem is in the swamps, you may tend to find demoralizing reasons for every good fortune that comes your way, with or without an effort on your part. Take my example as a model you shouldn't follow.

I get a fine job on an internationally known paper, and promptly some nasty little voice inside me begins to whisper that I got it by default. That is, this country's preparations for war had depleted the manpower pool, and employers like the *Wall Street Journal* were now willing to settle for guys like me. And when the chief of the copy desk pounced on my work, his angry criticisms ballooned my own feelings of inadequacy.

Ditto with my service in the air wardens. While my friends and relatives were able to risk their lives for their country, my disability provided me with a lame excuse for getting out of the draft.

Now how about seeing things another way, as I presently learned to do? When the tragedy of war created attractive openings for high-school graduates and even for dropouts like me, I was given a chance to try out for a job that would otherwise be closed to me, regardless of my ability. In this and many other ways my handicap proved to be an asset—nothing to be ashamed of. It had taken me many years of living with polio to come to terms with it and be gratified that I was given a chance.

Handicapped people everywhere have honed their abilities on misfortune. The media is rich with stories of disabled men and women who have amazed the world with their extraordinary achievements. One of them, within memory, became one of the greatest presidents this country has known. I am referring, of course, to Franklin Delano Roosevelt, who, like me, was a polio victim. What better role model can one ask?

TO PARENTS AND OTHER CONCERNED ADULTS: Telling a young person that his disability makes him unfit to hold a job may spring from a desire to protect him from the hard knocks of the world, which it certainly can do. But it can deliver a truly damaging blow to his self-esteem. If he is already coping with a damaged self-image, keeping him out of the work place could perpetuate his problem. It offers him a reason to avoid testing his adequacy.

I will not attempt to analyze my mother's motives. I am sure she had problems of her own in raising me, especially in light of Daddy O.'s reaction when I was stricken with polio: He fled. I am also sure that she wanted to protect me from risks, as she demonstrated when she took me out of a regular public school and put me into a class for the handicapped.

My own reaction to her declarations of my unfitness was to excuse myself from presenting myself physically to a world I feared. Instead, I felt justified in staying home, educating myself with books and talks with my educated friends, and putting all my energy into writing poetry. I soothed my ego with acceptances by respected magazines and newspapers, but nagged myself with the prospect of endless dependency on my mother.

Assurance that I would not be cruelly kicked around in the world of employment, that I could handle myself and perform any number of jobs besides writing poetry, would, I believe, have helped me to get on track many years earlier than I got there on my own. It might also have motivated me to continue my formal education so that I could wave a diploma at prospective employers.

There was scant literature on parenting in those days. Parents with special problems, like my mother, had to figure things out for themselves. And so did their handicapped children, whose guidance was mostly from their parents.

Even today many parents are confused about helping their youngsters, especially the handicapped, to a good start. I would certainly advise them (as you, patient reader, anticipate) to get professional counsel.

TO EMPLOYERS OF THE HANDICAPPED: There has been an upsurge of consciousness about the desirability of bringing handicapped people into the work force. And it has paid off. Many of them, motivated by a powerful need to show the world what they can do, make an extra effort to be outstanding employees.

If there is a handicapped person in your employ, and you're just a little uncomfortable about it, won't you please make an effort to examine your feelings. At some unconscious level you may be assuming that because his legs are paralyzed, his hearing, his eyesight, and his intelligence are also deficient. If you discover that you are talking to him in an extra-loud voice, for instance, or in an overexplanatory manner, ask yourself whether this is really called for.

And if you find yourself worrying about what impression your department will make on new accounts with a disabled employee in your midst, try to clarify this uneasiness in your mind. You will be getting in step with the new trend of recognizing the handicapped as a neglected minority. More than that, you will be overcoming a prejudice that limits your perceptions and may infect those around you.

CHAPTER
18

IF YOU CAN'T WALK, DRIVE!

My job on the *Wall Street Journal* gave me a welcome new feeling that maybe I could make it through life on my own. Coincidentally—or synchronistically—my mother obtained a transfer to a Brooklyn school. I announced that I wanted my own place, and she agreed that it might be a good idea.

I found a very cozy two-room apartment on the ground floor of what was once a private house, and with a feeling of anxious exhilaration, I moved in. I was on my way out of the stable.

I have already mentioned the excruciating self-consciousness I experienced walking on the streets of New York in the company of another conspicuously handicapped person. I used to feel that the sight of two of us together was sending out a message that we belonged in a separate compartment of the human race.

As I matured, I began to recognize the ridiculousness of my feelings, but my intellectual understanding was feeble in the face of the invading emotions. I admired the nonchalance of some of my handicapped friends when they walked with me; but much as I strove to emulate them, I could not master my queasiness—not until I got to know Danny Bloom.

I had moved from the *Wall Street Journal* to a better paying position on the copy desk of the *New York Herald Tribune*, a full-size paper that rated second only to the *Times*. Here, after a few days, I became acquainted with this friendly extrovert. Danny came to work in a wheelchair, which he used instead of a regular chair to sit at his place on the city desk. He was good medicine for me; simply by example he taught me that my handicap need not keep me out of highly respected positions or deplete the quality of my life.

Danny drove a car, and when I asked him how this was possible, he explained the mystery of hand controls and gave me the address of a company in New Jersey that installed them. He also gave me the name and address of a driving school that taught driving with hand controls. Finally he told me how to get a Special Vehicle Identification card that would give me special parking privileges in New York City.

Pretty soon I was taking the subway to Brooklyn for my driving lessons. My teacher was an alcoholic named Mickey, a street kid who, with the help of Alcoholics Anonymous, had pulled himself out of the gutter into a constructive way of life. He not only had a job, but was married and was the father of a small child. Mickey had been dry for about a year when I started lessons with him. He was big, lank, Irish, friendly, and wonderfully patient with me. In the course of our hours together we struck up a friendship that was to last a couple of years.

In a short time I passed my driving test, bought a car, had

it equipped with hand controls, procured my Special Vehicle Identification card and was driving ecstatically to work through the jungles of New York traffic. My mother cried throughout all this. She was sure I was going to kill myself. But I was beginning to be gung-ho about myself, and I felt nothing could stop me now.

On foot I had always drawn sympathetic glances, offers to help, and a feeling that I was one of God's inferior creations. In my little car, however, I felt like hell on wheels. No, I don't mean that I drove recklessly. I mean that when impatient drivers honked or shouted obscenities at me, as is the time-honored custom in New York City, it made me feel great; the car was in many ways like a new body; I could move as fast or as slowly or as skillfully as the next guy.

I am sorry to add that my instructor, a devout Catholic, fell off the wagon a few months after my driving lessons were terminated. In his cups, Mickey would call my home at all hours of the night and shout into the telephone a mixture of religion and profanity and love and hate. I would try to calm him down, and sometimes our talks would last for one or two hours. It was my first informal venture into offering talk therapy to a person in trouble. Perhaps I should say "listening therapy," for Mickey did most of the talking. He told me I was helping him, and I think this may have stirred some deep-down dream in me of becoming a real therapist.

I wish I knew where Mickey is today, and whether he has found the kind of help I could not offer him in the days before my training in therapy.

In the course of my driving lessons, Mickey introduced me to Saint Anthony, who is supposed to be the patron saint of sailors, but who may be willing to take on many other tasks—for a fee, according to Mickey; he confided that Saint Anthony "will do anything you ask if you promise him a quarter."

"How can you give him a quarter?" I wanted to know.

"Oh, you put it in the collection box next time you go to church."

I certainly had to test this out. That night I lost my watch, and promptly offered the good saint a quarter if he would help me find it. A few minutes later my eye caught sight of the watch on the floor. Coincidence? Well, I tested it out over and over and was amazed at how well it worked. Now and then it didn't, and I would wonder if I was pushing my connection too far.

I am not much of a churchgoer, so I found my own way of giving Saint Anthony his quarters. At the end of every month, I would make a contribution to some charity I felt partial to. Even today, my wife Gwen and I are still doing that—and it still seems to work. We never drive into Manhattan without asking Saint Anthony to find us a parking spot. And he does!

Years later a severe test of the good saint's ability to find a parking space for me came on Saint Patrick's Day. Though my car displays the police card I mentioned above, entitling me to park wherever the signs say, "No Parking," the parking rules in Manhattan are lifted on holidays.

By that time I was working as the senior editor of *Venture—The Traveler's World,* on Madison Avenue, within a couple of blocks of Saint Patrick's Cathedral—the very worst area to look for parking spaces on Saint Patrick's Day. I drove around for fifteen or twenty minutes and finally called on the saint for help.

A moment later I stopped for a red light right on the corner facing the cathedral. In front of me, in the middle of the intersection, I saw two police officers talking to each other. I gave a gentle honk on my horn and heard one of them say to the other, "Excuse me a minute while I take care of this V.I.P."

He strolled over to my window and asked, "What can I do

for you?" On an impulse I took my police card off the dashboard and handed it to him. My name, Garrett Oppenheim, was clearly typed on it.

"The name's O'pennim," I said, "and I need a parking place."

That very nice officer looked around carefully and pointed to a nearby space where someone was pulling out. "There you go," he said.

Don't tell *me* Saint Anthony's powers are all in my imagination!

I would like to insert a profound quote from the ancient Greek philosopher Hippocrates: "Prayer indeed is good, but while calling on the gods a man should himself lend a hand."

My reliance on Saint Anthony generated some new questions in my mind. I had seen a Goddess, and my prayers had always been addressed to her. Would she be angry and disown me if I kept petitioning the saint?

The question began to strike me as foolish. What knowledge I had accumulated about religions, plus my own experience, had led me to the obvious conclusion that God can be worshiped by any name or in many guises.

TO PARENTS: Conspicuous in the dreams of practically any kid is the image of himself at the wheel of a shiny car. To the handicapped kid, it can mean a lot more than that. The car doesn't have to be shiny, either. It just has to go.

If your handicapped son or daughter wants to learn how to drive, encourage him (or her) to get lessons, whether from a professional teacher or from a sympathetic friend. Even if it's impractical for your family to own a car, encourage him. One thing always leads to another. Once he develops the skill, chances are he'll get some kind of car in some way you may not have even imagined.

As you've seen in my case, just driving a car can bring about an extraordinary change in his feelings about himself. And when his dream of owning one comes true, he'll discover that a car makes friends. He'll be called on for favors and for help in emergencies. It can do a lot for his self-esteem. Instead of seeing himself as an outsider or, even worse, a drag, he has something to offer. It brings him into the fold.

TO THE HANDICAPPED: If you want to learn how to drive, remember that you have resources available to you. There are professional driving schools and even some rehabilitation centers (like the Helen Hayes Hospital in West Haverstraw, New York) that have specially equipped cars and instructors.

Take the lessons and get your driver's license. Even if it's impractical for you or your family to own a car, you will have proved to your parents, your friends, your employer, and— most important—yourself that you can do it. And, if you eventually do get a car, your boundaries will expand significantly.

As you've seen in my case, just driving gave an extraordinary boost to my feelings about myself. I made friends, I helped friends, and in many cases I changed the way others think about me—all thanks to this mechanical wonder.

If your parents feel too uneasy or will not give it their blessing, remember that it's important for you to do what you feel is right for you. Eventually you will be in complete control of your own life. The sooner you do what you can for yourself, the better off you will be in the long run, and the better you will feel about yourself.

CHAPTER
19

OPENING THE FLOODGATES

One afternoon as I was making my way into the city room of the *Herald Tribune*, I was approached by a man who walked with two crutches and wore a cast on one leg.

"I'm Jack Danby," he said. And without further introduction he explained that he'd taken a spill, broken his leg in two places and been forced to stay home for a week.

"I'm Garrett Oppenheim," I said. "I started work here as a copy editor a few days ago. I've heard stories about you. I gathered that you must be at least ten feet tall."

Jack laughed. Actually his stature, like mine, was well below average. By this time I was beginning to feel that a powerful kinship had sprung up between us. In the next few minutes we learned that we both had been hit by polio, that we were both copy editors, and that we wanted to be friends.

"Actually, I'm not as crippled as I look," Jack was eager to

explain. I put those words in italics, because I think they make a great statement—not only about Jack Danby, but about every handicapped person who has met the challenge that was imposed on him. In my eyes, Jack really was ten feet tall.

I learned that he could transform his physical disability into outstanding achievements on behalf of handicapped people everywhere. Another thing that impressed me was Jack's unquenchable sense of humor; he told terrible jokes, one after another in rapid succession. What Jack did for me was nothing short of remarkable. Let me be specific.

In those days we lived in the same neighborhood on the periphery of Columbia University, whose numerous buildings occupy several blocks. We also worked the same night trick on the paper, and we often rode the subway uptown together. Sometimes we'd stop off at the West End Cafeteria for a beer. More often we'd end up at my little apartment on 118th Street to have a drink or two and begin the long unwinding that every copy editor needs after the last deadline. Then I'd walk Jack back to his place for a few last snatches of friendly talk before turning in.

Imagine one of those soft summer nights when the small-hours' stillness seems to reach out and enfold you in serenity. Then picture the two of us, both mellow, limping along 116th Street, flanked on both sides by university buildings. All the sidewalks on Columbia property are paved with red bricks instead of smooth concrete.

Somewhere in the middle of the block, Jack spotted a big dolly—one of those low platforms on wheels that are used for moving heavy equipment. He gave it a playful poke with one of his canes.

The thing took off, weaving down the brick slope with an electrifying clatter—with two crippled copy editors in hot pursuit. The alarming thought had crossed both our minds that unless we could stop it, that damn fool dolly was going right on to Broadway and out into the traffic!

What a brave scene we must have made, limping along at high speed, our canes flying, our steel braces flashing in the lamplight under our trousers, and Jack muttering, "Son of a bitch! Son of a bitch!"

The runaway dolly was dangerously close to the intersection when we caught up with it. Jack was about to give it a nudge with one of his canes when the thing veered out of his reach and rumbled toward me. I gave it a vigorous poke with *my* cane.

That did it. The dolly swerved providentially into a brass standpipe and came to a stop. The great chase ended with the two of us leaning against a palace of learning, laughing and panting and bellowing like bulls.

It was a great moment in my life. I could actually feel the stigma, the disgrace, the self-imposed humiliation of a limp pouring out of my body on waves of laughter. From that night on, I knew, I could be what I am and who I am and take the whole big world into my heart.

My dear friend Jack Danby has passed on to another realm, but I will always be grateful to him for helping me break free from the prison of shame in which I had immured myself. I hope you can hear me, Jack, when I say "Thank you, thank you, thank you!"

TO THE HANDICAPPED: Stop worrying about the way other people see you and learn to enjoy just being whatever you are. That's pretty shopworn advice to give to anybody, but how many people follow it? In particular, how many handicapped people can act on it?

I'm painfully aware that some people don't see you as a card-carrying member of the human race, but you must constantly remind yourself that this is their problem, not yours. Once you release yourself from the feeling that their perception of you may have nothing to do with who you are, you can learn to laugh off your own insecurities. I mean really laugh them off. Your life should be fun!

Modern scientists and writers such as Norman Cousins and Bernie Siegel have been affirming what primitive peoples knew long ago—that you can't feel depressed while you're having fun. As Edgar Cayce put it, " . . . the body . . . should be out-of-doors more; holler, yell more, for the fun of it!" (3564-1)

The Greeks knew this when they established their annual Dionysian festival, in which the whole population let their hair down and danced in the streets. In our present culture some people still find their outlets in slapstick comedies that invite them to identify with such classic pie-in-the-face comedians as the Marx Brothers and Lucy (Lucille Ball).

If you have been going through life with an exaggerated concern about your public image, my prescription is: Go crazy! Act wild! Let it all out! You may have a revelation about the divine sense of fun that lets us forget such picayune concerns as, "Is this the wrong necktie?" or "Is my color scheme obsolete?" or "Does my limp attract the wrong kind of attention?"

I know a dwarf woman with an ebullient personality, though she stands less than four feet high. At her sister's wedding reception, when the music started and the floor began to fill with dancing couples, this wonderful young woman caught the spirit, marched out onto the floor, and began dancing exuberantly all by herself. You could tell by her laughing eyes that she was dancing with a partner nobody else could see. It was a beautiful sight!

CHAPTER
20

AN INSTANT FAMILY

My first impression of Dona was that I was looking at a Greek statue. Her facial expression was slow to change and her marble-cool features seemed to inhibit conversation. We met at a small get-together in my home when her fiancé, a friend of ours, wanted to introduce her to my family. We all sat around rather stiffly, trying to manufacture small talk.

I didn't see Dona again for two or three years, when she and her two small children moved in with her parents. Their apartment was just a few blocks away from mine, and soon her parents invited me over for a great Italian dinner. I can only guess that their motive may have been to find company for their daughter. I began to be interested.

Dona apparently enjoyed talking with me. She didn't seem to mind that I wore a leg brace and walked with a cane. Nor did she seem to mind adjusting her pace to mine on the street. We had many outings together with the children, introducing them to the parks, the museums, the restaurants, the boat rides. I was working on the *Herald Tribune* at the time, and I took pleasure in showing them around the plant.

I fell in love with the children and became more and more involved with their mother, who was a keen observer and had many artistic talents. I soon learned that Dona's surface coolness masked a shaky self-esteem.

As the months went by I began to think that I might after all be capable of living a fulfilling family life. I began suggesting marriage, more and more insistently. Dona kept putting me off with such statements as, "I like you, but I just don't feel that way about you." And so I began to wonder: Was it the polio once more building a wall I could not seem to break through?

One day while we were walking with her children, Dona surprised me by saying simply, "I'll marry you." I gave her a big hug right there on the street.

At the same time, the thought of limping down the aisle with my bride on one side and my cane on the other held some psychological terrors for me. Suppose I should fall? I felt it would have permanently ruined the picture we all summon in our minds when we hear the word "wedding." And, of course, I could never carry the bride across the threshold.

I was relieved on learning that Dona didn't want any of that "claptrap." My feeling of being stigmatized, which had plagued me since childhood, was still there, but it was diminishing.

We asked a minister we knew to marry us in the chapel of his church in Brooklyn. I wanted a very private ceremony. My mother was rather opposed to the marriage, and I did not want her disapproving presence to put a damper on the occasion. If Dona's parents attended, my mother would be doubly hurt. So we decided to ask nobody.

However, my best friend in the air wardens insisted on coming. Warren pointed out that we needed a car, which he had, to get to the church, and a witness, which he would be. I consented gratefully.

We had found an apartment in the area where our two families were already living, and I began to feel that I was coming out of the swamps into an unbelievable paradise. The children, Karen and David, were easy to love, and I discovered that their curiosity about my lameness was more of a bonding factor than a dividing one. They asked many questions and sharpened my skill in answering.

I soon began to apply this skill in dealing with other children. Today, when a tot on the street asks her mother, "Why is that man walking funny?" and the mother in embarrassment starts to shush-shush the child and hurry away, I try to interrupt the ritual. I signal the mother to please not silence the kid. Then I speak to the little inquirer somewhat like this:

"You asked a very good question. Would you like me to tell you why I walk like this?"

The astonished child nods.

"When I was very little—littler than you—I got a sickness called polio. It stopped my legs from growing and getting strong, so now I use a cane to help me walk. This will never happen to you, because doctors have found a way to keep the sickness from coming to children. But I really don't mind walking funny, 'cause it makes children ask questions and I like to make friends with them."

If I get further questions, I try to answer them in kind. It is my hope that these children at least will grow up with a sense of understanding about the handicapped.

On weekends we usually visited my mother or my wife's parents. Dona's father had acquired a summer house on a woodsy property in Pearl River, New York, less than an hour from Manhattan. I hit it off fine with Homer, who was a professional carpenter, and we soon became very good friends.

Because I always had some writing project going and needed a quiet place to work, Homer built me a little one-room cabin in the woods on his property. Here I could spend productive hours at my typewriter or serene hours of meditation. Sometimes Dona and the children would come to the cabin for a quiet visit.

But early on, doubts began to creep in. We had started quarreling even before our marriage, and there were times when I wondered if we were doing the right thing for ourselves and the children. Our quarrels grew in frequency and intensity. Dona accused me of cheating, something I have never done. And I was always trying to keep the decibels down so the children wouldn't hear us.

I persuaded Dona to come to my therapist with me, but he apparently was not well schooled in resolving marital problems like ours. All he could offer us was Band-Aid® medicine. So the distance between us kept widening.

One day after a happy Chinese lunch, a quarrel erupted as we were all walking home. In the middle of it, Dona grabbed the two children by the hands and said, "Come on, let's get away from him." She began running ahead at a pace I had no way of keeping up with. The children kept looking back at me to see if I was catching up, but by the time I reached our building, they had already taken the elevator upstairs.

I felt that my wife was using my handicap to humiliate me and alienate the children. But I told myself that peace was my first priority, and I never brought up the subject. I knew that Dona was a good person, but I was finding out how a quarrel could wipe out that goodness and make her reach for any weapon to hurt. She went right for my most vulnerable point.

Some years later, when our marriage was in very turbulent waters, Dona fired this classic remark at me: "It's no fun being married to a cripple!"

The words burned into me, just as my father's poetry had done when I was ten years old. Only in this case the message was not subliminal; it was blatant.

Two weeks later, when Dona was freed of her overwhelming anger, she apologized. "I shouldn't have said that," she volunteered. But that didn't erase my conviction that this feeling was in her. I have never forgotten that blow to our marriage—or my self-esteem.

By this time our family had been augmented by the birth of a beautiful little girl, whose love for both of us helped to hold our marriage together. But it didn't hold for long. Presently I was living in a small apartment by myself, seeing the children on weekends.

TO ABLE-BODIED SPOUSES: It's so easy, when angers flare, to hit out at your spouse where you know it's going to inflict the deepest wound. And if your spouse happens to have a physical handicap, you've got an all-too-easy target. Sometimes the nicest people can't refrain from using it.

We are all familiar with the way schoolchildren can gang up on a vulnerable classmate and taunt him with such appellations as fatty, dirty Jew, runt, or whatever else may hurt the most. What we may not realize, and what we must be on guard against, is the fact that anger can regress us emotionally to childhood—the worst aspects of childhood.

Anger, even when justifiable, is always destructive. It can keep us awake nights while we go over and over the anger-generating scene. We agonize: I should have said this; I shouldn't have said that, and on and on. It saps the strength we could be using constructively.

Anger is contagious. It stirs gut emotions in others. If

reckless slurs are flung out in front of children, they can breed prejudice and hate. They can also drive a deep wedge into your relationship with the person you love.

When you feel the fiery flare of anger inside of you, that is the time to be especially wary of saying things you may later regret. Your words may be forgiven but not forgotten.

TO THE HANDICAPPED SPOUSE: If, in a bad moment, your partner uses your disability to wound you, try to understand that being married to you may be confronting her (or him) with some of the same problems you had to cope with in growing up: self-consciousness in public, restrictions as to what pleasures you can enjoy together, the knowledge that physically you are not exactly the idol of her teen-age dreams.

It may occur to you that your wife (or husband) has some problems of her own, such as low self-esteem, lack of social know-how, or inability to hold up her end of a conversation. This in turn may lead to the thought that she chose a handicapped partner because that might be all she could get.

Throw this idea right into the nearest garbage can! It denigrates the integrity of the partner you chose to live with. It plants the worms of doubt into your relationship.

The best way out, I have found, is to talk to her honestly about your own difficulty living in an impaired body and invite her to share her feelings on this subject with you.

Sometimes, in my opinion, divorce or separation may be the wisest answer, if only to protect the children from a tension-filled household. We all know that divorce is a deeply traumatic experience for the children. But living with quarreling or unhappy parents, as every therapist knows, can be much worse.

If divorce is decided on, it is important that the children be assured neither parent is abandoning them. Careful, repeated explanations are in order. Each child must know that he is not at fault for the split-up and that the parent who moves out will continue to be a good mother or father. Finally, each child must be convinced that he will have a happier home when there is no more quarreling between his parents.

Professional help is always desirable. Unfortunately, it is expensive, and it doesn't always work. Picking a therapist out of the telephone book is risky. It's usually a better idea to get a referral from a pediatrician or a hospital or some other trustworthy source.

CHAPTER
21

THE WEEKEND FATHER

Though I was extremely conscious of the dangers of favoring my own biological child over the two older ones, it was a danger hard to escape from. Karen and David had been through their mother's earlier divorce and seemed to be handling this second rift better than my daughter Lyn.

Hardest for me to cope with were Lyn's pleas for me to come home. Explain as I might, she would always respond, "I want you home, Daddy."

I tried to restore her spirits by taking her out on wonderful weekends. Since she had a passion for horses, I would drive her to a stable in Westchester to learn riding, English saddle. She fell in love with the horses and quickly became a very good equestrian. In her riding jacket and velvet cap and carrying a small riding crop, she loved to gad around town with me.

Among the highlights of our good times together were

our trips to Woodstock, New York. We spent many hours browsing in the fascinating shops and making occasional purchases.

Another favorite destination of ours was Stratford, Connecticut, the summer theater that featured Shakespeare's plays. Lyn quickly developed a love for the Bard. Before going to a play, we would spend an evening reading it. I would translate the Elizabethan English into modern American, and we had many good laughs over that. In *A Midsummer Night's Dream*, for instance, Shakespeare advises:

> Four days will quickly steep themselves in night;
> Four nights will quickly dream away the time . . .

Our translation: "Time flies."

And Hamlet's soliloquy—

> To be, or not to be: that is the question:
> Whether 'tis nobler in the mind to suffer
> The slings and arrows of outrageous fortune,
> Or to take arms against a sea of troubles,
> And by opposing end them? To die: to sleep;
> No more; and by a sleep to say we end
> The heartache and the thousand natural shocks
> That flesh is heir to . . .

Comes out: "Either I kill myself or I face my problems and put an end to them."

It was a fun game, and instead of putting the Bard down in her mind, it created a deep admiration for him and a lasting love for the beautiful poetry with which he could express the simplest of thoughts. Moreover, explaining Shakespeare to my daughter deepened my own appreciation of the Bard's profundity.

We went to the circus. We went to the movies. We shopped. We watched television together, especially the Flintstones.

Though we were living hand-to-mouth, there came a Christmas when I stumbled on a bonanza of gifts that I was able to shower on the three children. One of the reporters on the *Herald Tribune* covered the toy market and asked me to make a list of what the kids wanted Santa Claus to bring them. (This was a perfectly acceptable practice in those days, though today I think it would be severely frowned upon.) Lyn's list was formidable. I explained to her that she might get one or maybe two of the items on her sheet.

On Christmas morning I picked Lyn up after she had celebrated with her mother. When we arrived at my apartment, she made a dash to our little tree to see which items on her list might be under it.

She was overwhelmed. Not one, not two, but all the presents she had listed were there. But the gift that really excited her was a little packet of fifty-two cards that I had cut out of cardboard. On each card I had written, "Good for one Jeannie story." She still remembers that as "the nicest Christmas present I ever had."

Who was Jeannie? She was a mischievous little girl, just about Lyn's age, who had her own devious ways of setting wrongs to right. She was born, full blown, from my imagination while we were driving home from a day in the country.

Jeannie had friends from the other realm—elves and fairies, spirits who had magical powers and were able to share them with this special little girl. Jeannie could levitate and fly, she could use a certain ring one of her otherworld friends had given her. It enabled her to see what other people had in their pockets. She usually carried an arsenal of unusual weapons in her own pockets.

There was always a hopeless situation and neither Lyn

nor I ever knew how Jeannie was going to get out of it until some happy solution just seemed to come to me.

What was Jeannie's charm? I had no idea at the time, but I was a bit worried about the degree to which her outlawed escapades intrigued my daughter. So I made up a story telling how Jeannie was taken to a psychiatrist and began to enjoy a whole new kind of life as a "good girl." She learned how to make floral bouquets for her classroom. She volunteered to run errands for her parents. She threw away all the weaponry in her pockets. And so on.

This lasted for not quite two Jeannie stories. Toward the end of the second one, Lyn interrupted and said, "Daddy, tell me a story about Jeannie before she went to the psychiatrist."

Today, as a psychotherapist, I would guess that Jeannie was a kind of shadow personality who unleashed into an acceptable channel all sorts of unacceptable, suppressed feelings in my daughter—and maybe in me! After all, Jeannie was the creation of *my* inner mind.

A child who is coping with a lot of anger will often create fantasies of supernatural powers that enable her to deal with her fears—fears of ostracism, of abandonment, of physical harm. Many grown-ups do the same, only the content and characters in their fantasies may be different from those of a child.

Children are quick to anger, but generally have neither the power nor the permission to express it. It can build up huge tensions in their psyches and create behavior problems that can last a lifetime.

My daughter Lyn, I know, was full of anger in her childhood—at me, at her mother, at her siblings, her teachers, and schoolmates. She was also full of passionate love, and I can only guess at the inner conflicts she experienced. The Jeannie stories, depicting a little girl with supernatural powers that enabled her to conquer her fears, must have provided the channel she needed, for they seemed to be a very important part of her inner life.

In the midst of a heated quarrel she would suddenly pull out a Jeannie ticket and hand it to me. The message was unmistakable, and it generally cleared the air. The stories I created for her were hardly masterpieces, but they did seem to fulfill a therapeutic need.

INTERLUDE: A JEANNIE STORY

Jeannie had a dream one night—well, it wasn't really night; it was around six o'clock in the morning, she figured, because the dream made her jump out of bed and look at the clock. It said seven minutes after six.

The dream was about Mitch, one of her classmates, who was also one of her very best friends. Someone was chasing him, and when they came to a big, high cliff, that someone was just about to push Mitch over it. That's when Jeannie jumped out of bed and pulled on her clothes. She knew that she had some important work to do for her friend Mitch.

"I've got to be ready," she told herself. She began stuffing her pockets—she had an awful lot of pockets—with a bunch of things that were on the table next to her bed—three little artificial wiggly worms that looked very real, a little bag filled with itching powder, a big, ugly black spider that could crawl when you gave it a squeeze, four stink bombs, a make-believe cigarette, a rubber dagger, a shock stick, and a blond wig—just in case.

When she was all dressed and ready, Jeannie went to the window and opened it. She stuck her head out a little and called softly, "Galina, are you there?"

There was a gust of wind that sent the curtains flying to the ceiling. A beautiful fairy who looked like a princess came gliding through the window and touched down right in front of Jeannie. Waving her sparkling wand, she said, "You have a real hard job ahead of you, so I'm going to give you a special gift." She put a silver ring on the middle finger of Jeannie's right hand. "When you give this ring a little turn to the left," she said, "you will become completely invisible—you and all your clothes and all the things you have in your pockets."

"Oh, thank you, Galina!" Jeannie whispered. But Galina had already disappeared.

Three hours later Jeannie was sitting in her classroom. She wasn't paying as much attention as she knew she should to Miss Clark, the teacher. Miss Clark was talking about ancient history, which was not one of Jeannie's favorite subjects.

In the row ahead of her was her friend Mitch, and two seats away from him, right in front of Jeannie, was a boy named Clancy. He was the biggest boy in the class, and the other kids were all afraid of him. He would pick fights that he knew he would win. One time he had pulled Jeannie's hair so hard that she screamed.

Jeannie suddenly realized that Clancy was the one in her dream who had chased Mitch to the edge of the cliff, so she decided to get to work right away. She opened her bag of itching powder and carefully poured a little of it onto a ruler. Then, when Miss Clark was writing on the blackboard, Jeannie gently blew the itching powder at Clancy's neck.

After a minute or two, Clancy began to squirm in his chair. While he was squirming, Mitch raised his hand and asked to leave the room. When Clancy saw this, he asked to leave the room, too. And Jeannie knew she had to act quickly.

She gave her silver ring a little twist to the left, and didn't feel anything happening. She could still see her hands, her clothes, and everything. So she raised her hand. Nobody seemed to notice. Jeannie stood up. Still, nobody noticed. So Jeannie tiptoed out of the room. As she was leaving, she heard Miss Clark saying, "Anybody know what happened to Jeannie?"

Jeannie raced to the boys' room. She knew she wasn't allowed to go in, but this was an emergency. So in she went. And she didn't like what she saw. Mitch was trying to get out, but Clancy had grabbed one of his arms and was twisting it.

Jeannie already had her shock stick in her hand. She came up silently behind Clancy and touched his neck with it.

Clancy let go of Mitch's arm and turned around quickly to see who did that. He looked confused—and a little scared. While he was trying to figure things out, Mitch let him have a punch in the ribs. Clancy ran out as fast as he could. But Jeannie ran right after him and followed him right back into the classroom. He was panting so hard that Miss Clark asked him, "Are you all right, Clancy?"

Before he could answer, Jeannie let him have another shock in the neck. Clancy let out a yell and started for the door again. At the same time, Jeannie threw a stink bomb at the door. The class went crazy. Miss Clark quickly tied a handkerchief over her nose and mouth and shouted, "Class dismissed!"

As the class raced through the door, Jeannie saw Mitch coming out of the boys' room. Clancy saw him at the same time and began running after him. The whole class then started running after Clancy. They made such a racket that the school's fire alarm came on, and the whole school was racing to get out.

Jeannie, who was still invisible, was running as hard as she could because she knew what would happen. She had seen it in her dream. Clancy was going to push Mitch over the cliff unless somebody could stop him.

Clancy could run faster than Mitch because he was bigger and had longer legs. Jeannie was much smaller than both of them, and just couldn't catch up. She called in a scared whisper, "Help me, Galina! Help me quick!"

Jeannie was suddenly swept off the ground and lifted into the air and carried forward. She was set back down on the ground right at the edge of the cliff, but turned around so that she faced all the running kids. Unless she did something quickly, she would be pushed right over.

"Worms!" she heard Galina whispering in her ear. She reached into her pocket and came up with three wiggly worms. She shouted, "Look out, Mitch!"

Mitch heard her and realized that he was at the edge of the cliff. He turned and ran to the left. Clancy came to the edge of the cliff, panting hard, with his mouth wide open. Jeannie didn't think twice. She just slapped him across the lips, leaving his mouth full of worms.

Clancy stopped cold. He began spitting onto the ground. And when he saw what came out of his mouth, he leaned over and threw up. All the kids from the school were crowding around and laughing at him.

Jeannie gave her ring a turn to the right, and another great shout went up: "There's Jeannie!"

Mitch came over to Jeannie and gave her a big hug. "You saved my life," he said. And turning toward the crowd, he held one of Jeannie's arms up in the air. "She saved my life!"

Jeannie smiled one of her sweetest smiles. "That's what friends are for," she said.

CHAPTER
22

THE FULL-TIME FATHER

Because Lyn was too young to visit me by herself and because my tiny apartment could not sleep all three children, I found myself in some difficult situations. Lyn at her own request liked to stay overnight, and I was able to fix up a room for her. Finally she begged to live with me. I found a larger apartment for us on 12th Street, right next to a school that her mother and I both wanted her to attend. With Dona's consent Lyn moved in with me.

I had moved from the *New York Times* to *Medical Economics,* a prestigious magazine for physicians, which was located in Oradell, New Jersey. I would drop my daughter at school and then drive across the river to get to my job. As usual, problems came creeping in.

Lyn wanted me with her around the clock. Though I tried my best to help her understand the necessity of my working and her learning, the explanations didn't work.

She developed a school phobia.

No sooner did I get to my office in Oradell, than she would be on the phone with me from our apartment. She would plead illness or say that someone was "mean to me" or that I must come right home because the doorman had threatened her. I made innumerable trips across the Hudson River to allay her fears.

My production at work went down, and I began to get notes from the editor. I tried to catch up by working nights at home, but my daughter kept demanding attention from me. The editor gave me a deadline to pick up on my work or be dismissed.

I took Lyn to a professional therapist, who helped a lot. My work began to pick up. A copy girl who had access to the editor's desk confided that the editor had made himself a note to fire me unless . . . but then she gave me periodic reports that he was upgrading me. Soon after that she told me my rating was "Great!"

Lyn's teacher held conferences with me, and finally I was notified that my daughter could not reregister for the next term; her problems were too much for the faculty to handle. After a three-way conference with her therapist and Dona, and several talks with Lyn herself, we all agreed that she would be better off living with her mother. Dona was a full-time homemaker and could give Lyn the attention she needed.

Of course, I assured Lyn that I loved her as much as ever and that we would continue to have great weekends together. I told her that now she would have her mother to pick her up at school and spend time with her. There would be no more long hours alone at home. With all her unhappy experiences behind her, I think she understood me. But I was not surprised that she seemed very angry with me for a week or two. Though she didn't talk about it, I think she may have wondered whether I was abandoning her.

All through this period, Lyn's troubles had precluded any

kind of social life for me. I tried several times to resolve this situation by accepting invitations from friends. But early in the evening I would get a call from my daughter or her sitter to summon me home because things were not going well.

With Lyn's departure I began to pick up on my work and, to a small extent, on my friendships. Once more my weekends and vacations with Lyn resumed. They stand out as highlights for that period.

There has always been a powerful, intense bond between us—so powerful that I often wonder if our relationship harks back to a previous incarnation. Perhaps in that past lifetime we had problems with each other that were never worked out. Could that be why we have been brought together in this life—for another chance?

I am happy to report that Lyn finally emerged from her mixed-up childhood as a very beautiful, outgoing personality, with many talents that she is able to express—in the arts, in her career, in her friendships, and, most important, in love.

———

TO PARENTS: If you believe, as I do, in the concept of reincarnation and the laws of karma, you may well see a logical explanation of the difficulties that develop among individuals who are important to each other in the present life.

Under the laws of karma, as I understand them, if you had a relationship problem in some previous life and that problem was not resolved by the time of your death, you will have it all over again in a subsequent life. And if you don't want to have it plague you in one incarnation after another, you had better put your energy into resolving it now.

Let's presume that Lyn had some right to hold a grievance against me in another life. In this life we love each
other deeply, but that old grievance is, I would guess, now
lodged in her subconscious mind, which, as theorists tell
us, remembers everything. We have no way of knowing for
sure whether this theory is true, but there is a great body of
evidence to support it. Assuming it to be true, it would help
to explain Lyn's apparent fear that I would abandon her.

I would ask all parents, and specifically those who are
parents of the handicapped, to consider this explanation. It
can go far to help you understand some other inexplicable
behaviors of a troubled child. It certainly doesn't elucidate
everything, but often it can put your relationship in a new
light.

You might go further by asking a past-life therapist to take
you or preferably your child back to the life in which her
feelings about you had their source. As a therapist, I have
seen many puzzling behaviors change dramatically when
this source is unearthed. I make no claim for the literal au-
thenticity of regressions obtained in hypnosis, but I do
know that they can produce results.

If you do not believe in reincarnation or you do not see
your way clear to taking your child to a past-life therapist, at
least open your mind to the possibility of a karmic explanation. That alone could relax much of the tension between
the two of you. It might even put you and your child on the
road to a solution.

School phobia could be connected to the same symp-
tom—the fear of losing you. In any case it is a sticky kind of
fear that usually calls for skilled professional help. The
child's relationship with the parent or parents should be
thoroughly explored by a therapist.

If one of the parents is handicapped, it is quite possible
that his disability has something to do with the situation
that generated the problem. For instance, the image of "my

Daddy" that the child presents to her friends and class-mates may be one that she has been teased about. The child may then want to flee the classroom to her home. This and many other questions should be raised in the therapist's office.

CHAPTER
23

AN OLD GIRL FRIEND STEPS IN

As my career picked up, so did my social life. I was offered a very desirable position as senior editor of a new magazine called *Venture—The Travelers' World.* It was still not quite the kind of work I wanted to do, but it came a lot closer. The brilliant editor-in-chief, a soft-spoken, delightful man named Curt Anderson, gathered a staff of beautiful people to put together this very elegant magazine.

Before long I was driving four or five co-workers to restaurants in the countryside for evenings of socializing. I soon realized how much I needed grown-up people around me—something I had missed during my complete absorption with my daughter. I was also able to renew my connections with long-lost friends and relatives. It was a good life, but I still had a nagging feeling that I was traveling on a wrong road. I wanted to be doing something that would help people.

Another one of those "coincidences" that seem to pop up throughout my life brought me a letter from California—from Fae, an old sweetheart from my youth.

Fae explained that she had been happily married to a kind and loving man for many years, but that he had died a year ago. While shopping in San Francisco, she had stopped at a pay phone to call a friend. She noticed a Manhattan directory in the booth, and the thought came to her: "I wonder if Garrett's number is still in the book?" She looked. It was. She wrote me a letter.

After a brief correspondence, Fae proposed using her vacation for a trip East to spend a couple of weeks with me. I had mixed feelings about that. On the one hand, I remembered those great evenings when we would read together or go out together. I remembered the daylong outings we enjoyed together, and many other happy moments.

On the other hand, I had been nursing a grudge all these years over an incident that happened long ago with her. I wondered if I could forgive and forget. It seems trivial now as I think about it, but at the time I was completely deflated over it.

I had two tickets for what I felt would be the concert of concerts—Toscanini, my favorite conductor, and Heifitz, my favorite violinist, and the great New York Philharmonic in a concert that featured Brahms's Violin Concerto, Brahms being my favorite composer at the time. I invited Fae to share this once-in-a-lifetime experience with me, even though I knew that she was not a lover of classical music. She accepted the invitation readily, and I was looking forward to the event in a state that bordered on delirium.

A couple of days before the concert Fae phoned to cancel the date with me. An old boyfriend from Canada, she explained, was going to be in New York that day, and she didn't want to miss seeing him.

I felt completely deflated. There was no one else I wanted

to take to that concert. I told Fae she could have the tickets so she and her friend would have a place to go. She accepted my offer gratefully, and I kicked myself for years after that.

Since this turn of events was completely my own doing, I had no reason to hold a grudge against Fae for all this time. In her position I am sure I would have done the same. But there it was.

Even though I felt awkward about spending my vacation with a woman I hardly knew after all these years, when she phoned and persisted, I couldn't resist her. After all, I was due for a vacation myself and had not yet decided how to use it.

I had just edited an article describing the beauties of Hilton Head Island, which writers and travel agents had discovered, and I decided to take Fae there by car. She flew from California and I met her at the airport. She was still the attractive woman I remembered.

It was early in the day, so I suggested that we head right out toward our destination. On the drive we began to catch up on all the events we each had experienced over these many years.

As we drove on, I brought up my memory of that night we had spent together on Hunter Island. Fae remembered it clearly, too. I couldn't help asking her: "Why did you keep pushing me off like that?"

Her response: "I felt you were just too immature."

It was as if something that had been constricting my chest all these years suddenly came undone and vanished. It wasn't my lame legs that had put Fae off—just my immaturity. I wondered silently how many other times in life I had been mistakenly sure that other people's reactions to me were based on my handicap. Fae's words told me by implication that things could be different now.

Along the way, after getting tired and hungry, we decided to take a room. I had not enjoyed any intimacy with a woman since Dona and I had split. And now, here I was in a strange hotel room, wondering what would happen next. The answer was ambiguous: We fell asleep in each other's arms. I wondered if this was going to be a friendly, innocent jaunt, like our canoe trips in the old days, or if we were going to have an affair.

We stopped at another motel for the night, and I soon had a much clearer answer. While we were unpacking, Fae began to talk about moving to New York and about the prospects of our marriage. I was completely taken aback. After my first experience with matrimony, I told her, I had no desire to tie the knot around me again—at least not for a while. But not knowing what I really wanted, I suggested that we go to bed and sleep on it.

The rest of the trip was a pleasant experience for both of us. I enjoyed being with a woman again. Fae was certainly a beautiful and loving person; but even though I felt very lonely, I had strong reservations about marriage. By the time we got back to New York, however, I found myself talking about shopping for wedding bands. Neither of us wanted a fancy ceremony.

It was a City Hall ceremony that took about five minutes, after which I brought my bride to *Venture's* office to introduce her to my colleagues. In no time at all they came up with a party for us. I was still too dazed to know how I felt about all this. Up until now I had really been enjoying my freedom.

Fae and I were hardly settled down in my apartment when *Venture* ceased publication. That very special magazine was part of the Cowles empire, publishers of *Look* and other popular magazines. The whole Cowles establishment was then in a state of collapse. The magazines were dying one by one, and when our turn came I discovered that after seven years on this job I was left with a lifelong pension of exactly $31.14 a month.

A few days after our farewell party at *Venture*, I found myself thinking that this misfortune might really be a great opportunity for me to live the kind of life of which I had always dreamed. I stepped up my writing again. By now I had published articles in *Cosmopolitan, Good Housekeeping, Women's Day,* and numerous other magazines. I was beginning to feel that I could take a chance on free-lancing.

But Fae, who was holding down a job herself, kept urging me to look for something steady and reliable. Half-heartedly, I applied at two places where I had already worked—at *Medical Economics,* which now had a more friendly editor-in-chief, and at the *New York Times.*

One day brought me job offers from both of those attractive publications. I found the idea of going back to either of them acutely depressing. I told Fae I wanted to turn them both down.

Fae said I was crazy to even think of passing up this chance for a secure income. She wanted to look forward to a retirement that eliminated chance. The idea of a free-lancing husband went entirely against the grain with her. After much discussion, I felt that while I was more than willing to take my own chances as a free-lance, I could not foist this insecurity on my wife.

Medical Economics and I got along just fine this second time around. Lyn seemed to be doing well in therapy, and I was no longer so totally sidelined by my consuming preoccupation with her problems. She was still a weekend guest, and our lives at this point seemed relatively storm-free.

On the other hand, I found myself experiencing little episodes of silent anger at Fae. Though I knew I had no right to blame her for talking me into a life that I considered nonproductive, I knew at another level that I was merely passing the buck. The truth was that we had different priorities. My deepest wish was to make some kind of contribution. Fae had always dreamed of security. Moreover, I was well aware that I had plenty of faults and that Fae was not backward in finding them out and urging me to change my ways.

On my part I found plenty of opportunities to channel my discontent into trivia. We seemed to be quarreling incessantly, and in the middle of our quarrels I would often forget what we were quarreling about.

I had been through enough psychotherapy to question myself, and I presently realized that the real target of my anger was me. I was angry at myself for not having enough respect for my own wishes and talents, for letting myself be led into somebody else's way of life without even finding a middle road.

I could also understand Fae's wish for financial security; she had been raised in an extremely impoverished household and had made her way alone in New York from the age of seventeen, holding thankless office jobs. I tried, then, to count my blessings.

Respecting my background and interests, Al Vogl, the editor-in-chief of *Medical Economics,* put me in charge of the division concerned with doctor-patient relations, family relations, psychosomatic illnesses, and the like. In a small way, I could be of some service here. At the same time, I was working for a magazine that insisted on clear, concise writing, and I was sharpening my skills in this field.

Fae and I moved to Tappan in Rockland County, just about thirty minutes out of New York City and fifteen minutes from my job. As a born New Yorker, I was pleased to see trees and flowers all around us and lots of sky unimpeded by any tall buildings. I wondered whether Manhattan's nervous energy was so deeply ingrained in me that I would feel lost. But Manhattan was only a short ride away, so we could still visit our old friends there or take in plays and museums. I have never regretted that move.

———

TO THE HANDICAPPED: Earning a living versus doing your own thing, these are two clashing maxims in the American psyche, and between my two daddies I had been brainwashed with both. I'm sure they pose an equally tough dilemma for many talented and spiritual individuals.

The chancy way to go is with Maxim Number One: "Be your own person and do your own thing." Maxim Number Two counsels prudence: "Face up to your responsibilities as a provider and build a comfortable nest for your family."

I was already quite pleased with what I had managed to achieve in spite of my handicap and my feelings about it. Could I bring myself to throw all that away and pursue a new, unknown path? Wouldn't that be pushing my luck? On the other hand, as an individual on a spiritual quest, would I be building myself a prison by positioning myself in the marketplace?

It's a very important question and, therefore, a very difficult one. And since each of us is an individual with a given set of strengths and since each of us is subjected to a special set of pressures, I certainly would not presume to tell any reader which way to go. I can only draw your attention to some points to consider.

In addition to that, I can tell you my own belief, based on my experience and the experiences of my patients: I believe in destiny and I believe in choices. In other words, when you must choose between two roads that take different directions, either road will lead you to the destination you were meant to get to. One road may be longer or harder than the other, but it will surely take you to the same place.

I have another belief that modifies what I have just said: You can just cop out. You can take no road and never arrive at your destination in this life. But my belief in reincarnation and the testimony of patients I have regressed to previous lifetimes tell me that if you fall short of your goals in this life, it's O.K.; you will have another chance next time around.

So if I have any advice to you, my handicapped reader, it can be put very simply: Size up the alternatives presented to you the best you can, then make your decision and trash your doubts. When you reach a point where you can look back on the road traveled, I think you will not regret your choice.

CHAPTER
24

LIFE TAKES A U-TURN

It was in the peaceful milieu of Tappan that I set my sights on the kind of life I had always wanted, a life in which I could help other people—and myself—to deeper levels of understanding. My own search had already led me to the conviction that every individual has within himself, at some level, the keys to resolving his own problems. I wanted to find a way to help others find those keys. I began to make my goals a little more specific and to develop some new ideas—new at least to me.

I felt I had enough experience and training—through my eleven years as a patient in psychoanalysis, through my years with my father and all his patient explanations, through the many books I had studied and digested, and through the articles I had researched and written in this field—to pursue my dream. I could offer friendly counsel to people who needed help, something on the order of

"Dear Abby" or "Ann Landers."

My idea was to set up a service in which I could counsel clients by mail or phone or on tape. We could do this evenings and sometimes on weekends, thus satisfying Fae's need for security and my own desire to be of service to people. Fae was fully supportive of the idea; so in 1971, with the assistance of a lawyer friend, we founded a small organization and named it Confide—Personal Counseling Services, Inc.

I took a mental inventory of my blessings: I am married to the girlfriend of my youth, and I am holding a very nice job as a senior editor of *Medical Economics.* Because of my own background and interest in psychology, I am often sent out to conferences and for interviews with leading authorities in this field. The important message to me in my inventory of blessings was that my physical handicap had never stood in the way of my getting the kind of assignments I wanted or in carrying them out. I felt I was transcending my handicap.

I liked journalism and enjoyed the perceptive people I met in the course of my duties, but it was not quite my thing. I had felt trapped in it for many, many years. Now I wanted to meet people on a one-to-one basis, to explore the inner mind. I sensed that somehow my plan would lead me deeper into the metaphysical world. And at this juncture I was beginning to put away my timidity about going after what I wanted out of life.

Meanwhile, I was studying evenings at home to work toward a doctoral degree in psychology. I felt I needed this not just for credibility but for honing whatever skills I had. Though I had not completed high school, I had done a great deal of post-graduate-level studying and writing.

With a little inquiring I discovered the many universities that offer home-study courses. The leading institution in this field, according to my research, was Columbia Pacific University.

C.P.U. accepted me on the basis of my writings and my experience. The story of my own psychoanalysis, which had been published in three installments in a magazine called *Why*, now extinct, was accepted as a Ph.D. thesis.

Armed with my plan and my ambition, I requested a four-day week at *Medical Economics* and rented a small office in Manhattan, where I could sit down with troubled clients on my days off and listen to them and perhaps offer some friendly counsel.

Almost immediately, I drew a client whose needs called for knowledge that was way over my head. He was a transsexual, a man who had a burning conviction that he was really a woman trapped in a male body.

Hardly anybody in those days even knew the word "transsexual," and I had no idea where to refer my client. I did know that many transsexuals were treated as psychotics, but I felt this was wrong. I started to search for someone who had expertise in this field, and my efforts soon brought me into a meeting with a remarkable physician. Harry Benjamin, the world's top authority on transsexualism, was eighty-nine years old at that time and still practicing on a limited scale.

My first meeting with him left me dazzled; I knew that I could learn important things from this wise pioneer. Over the next decade he became a close friend and mentor. I visited his home in downtown Manhattan once a week and plied him with questions or just listened to him. What he gave me was more valuable than a postgraduate course; it was advanced training, not only in the facts about transsexualism, but in the healing magic of empathy.

One day, as Harry was approaching his hundredth birthday, he told me he knew that his death was not far off. I asked him what he believed happens after death. "It's the end," he said. "We turn into dust." And he snapped his fingers by way of emphasis.

I told Harry that I believed in some kind of afterlife—that maybe we come back to earth for another chance to grow. Harry just shook his distinguished head and said, "Well, if I'm around, I'll let you know."

Harry Benjamin died at the age of 101, leaving a legacy that continues to bring peace and well-being to thousands of men and women who feel that they were born into the wrong bodies. He had told his wife and all his friends that he wanted his body to be cremated, and he definitely did not want a funeral. Instead, his friends got together for a meeting to exchange memories of Harry and his great contributions to humanity. Because I was privileged to be one of his friends, I was invited to be one of the speakers.

In the course of my talk I mentioned our conversation on death and its aftermath, and Harry's promise to let me know if he was still around. I had hardly got the words out of my mouth when, for no observable reason, the smoke alarm over my head came to life with a loud blast.

Coincidence? I knew better. I sent up a silent "Thank you, Harry!" and went on with my talk.

Long before I started my practice as a psychotherapist, I became interested in the concept of reincarnation. The idea of living just once, working and striving and finally being cut off by annihilation in death, seemed to me to take all the meaning out of life, out of striving, out of growth.

I like the idea of coming back again and again, each time—we hope—with more understanding. This concept gives me a reason to improve myself right up to the very moment of death. Worrying about the terrible mistakes I've made in this life seems contraindicated; if I can learn from them, perhaps I can move ahead to greater challenges in the next life.

Even if I go right on repeating my mistakes in this life, the next incarnation may give me another chance to correct them. Relationships that never worked out for me might, perhaps, be resolved beautifully next time around. We all know how nature renews itself with the seasons. Why not humankind?

The concept of synchronicity—the idea that when you are ready, the right events happen—keeps growing on me. I will tell a woman patient who is desperately lonely, "When you are emotionally ready, the right man will be there." He always is.

Three chance meetings ("chance," did I say? I'll never believe they were chance) pointed me in a new direction. The first was with Zelda Suplee, who has since passed on.

Zelda, another admirer of Harry Benjamin's, looked me up when she heard that I was working with transsexuals, a field in which she had a good deal of expertise. We soon became fast friends. We would meet whenever she was in New York to discuss our work and our beliefs.

Zelda liked to regress her friends to past lives as a hobby. She had attracted some notice when one of her subjects in hypnotic regression turned out to be a passenger on the Titanic when that great ocean liner went down. In his sessions with Zelda he was able to recapture vivid memories of those historic moments.

It was not surprising that we found each other at a national conference of the Harry Benjamin Gender Dysphoria Association, an organization of professionals who treat transsexualism. During a free evening, Zelda asked me if I would like her to take me into a past life. "I would love that," I said, and we went to her hotel room for quiet.

Zelda did a very brief induction, as the initial process of inducing a trance is called, and before I even felt that I was in an altered state, she asked me where I was. It was all very weird to me.

I found myself sitting in a box at the opera somewhere in Italy with a young woman. I had a sort of olive complexion, slicked black hair, and a small, agile-looking build. My companion, whom I hardly knew, had a creamy white skin, which gave her bare shoulders a sensuous appearance. She was richly dressed and looked the way I felt—bored!

As I gazed at her, I was thinking: When the opera is over, I will take her to a fancy little restaurant I know, and in the course of a platitudinous conversation we will learn a few superficial facts about each other. After that, we will go to my apartment, have a drink or two, and go to bed together. I had done this so many times with so many different women that I was hardly thrilled by the idea of going through the same old routine again.

While I was absorbed in these dreary thoughts, Zelda woke me up and questioned me about the regression. I told her the scene and finished with, "I guess I was a sort of arrogant snob in that life." I think I sounded disappointed. Privately, I was wondering if the scene had any validity. It was a question I couldn't answer.

Zelda asked me if I would like to try again, and I think I was eager to produce something a little more gratifying. She put me under hypnosis once more, this time somewhat deeper.

I found myself floating in the air over a dreary swamp at twilight. My first thought was, "What the hell am I doing up here?" Then I began to wonder, "Am I dead?"

I was floating toward land, and now I could see, off to one side, a brown structure in the shape of a Quonset hut. The end that was visible was all open—no door or wall to it. And emanating from the open space was a soft yellow light. I decided to investigate.

"If that's an electric light," I was thinking, "then this whole thing is a fraud." I floated myself somehow right into the structure, which was open at the other end as well.

I have only a hazy picture in my mind of the source of the light, but I could see that it came from small flames—candles or oil lamps, maybe. But what really caught my eye as I looked below was what appeared to be a dead body.

It was the body of a young woman, quite beautiful, light-skinned, dressed in clothes that made her look like an island princess. She was laid out on some kind of couch or table, and then apparently left there for the night.

Who might this lovely woman be? I floated down closer.

"It's me," I suddenly realized. And on the heels of that discovery a crazy idea hit me: What would happen if I got back into that body and sat up?

It was easy to let myself dissolve into the young woman's attractive body and begin to feel both my importance and my beauty. In a spirit of fun I swung my legs over the side of the couch and sat up. Almost immediately I could feel a living presence in the hut. It was a disapproving presence.

I don't argue with the gods. I pulled my legs up again and laid my body back down just the way I had found it. I was quite unhappy at being awakened by Zelda at this juncture.

Those two brief regressions stirred all sorts of fantastic ideas in me. Was it really possible to go back to another lifetime in hypnosis? Or did I make it all up? As I went on with my waking life, those questions receded into the back of my mind. But an incident in my office brought them back full force.

I had been working with a severely depressed client who had very violent fantasies. Sometimes he acted out his fantasies with the street gang to which he belonged. One night Les came to my office in a particularly severe state of depression. We decided to look for the source of these feelings, which we expected to find in some childhood trauma.

When I saw that Les was in a fairly deep state of hypnosis, I decided to take this very direct approach: "I'd like you to go back to the very first time in your life that you ever had this kind of feeling." Only I left out the words "in your life."

There was a long pause before I asked Les where he was.

"I'm on a battlefield," he said. "There are thousands of men in armor."

Further questioning revealed that Les was one of Hannibal's lieutenants fighting the Romans. He knew that he was going to win this battle, but he also knew that the Romans were going to win the war. Moreover, one of his aides, who was also his lover, had just broken up with him. They were apparently linked in some kind of gay relationship.

When I roused Les, his depression had lifted a good deal. In our subsequent discussion, so many new avenues of healing had opened up that Les's problem began to dissolve. This unexpected and astonishing result made me begin to think that past-life regression might be a wonderful pathway to healing.

I tried using past-life therapy with a few special patients, after discussing it with them and getting their permission. Consistently, I found I was getting better results with it than with more conventional approaches. I confess that I never felt sure my patients were telling me about actual events that happened long before they were born. Part of me believed, and part of me didn't.

The part of me that didn't believe came up with another theory: Perhaps these alleged past lives were metaphors that explained the patient's problems. In some cases, just reliving those past lives immediately eliminated such symptoms as phobias, performance anxieties, and compulsive behaviors. In others, they explained the troubles my patients were having, such as low self-esteem or difficulties in their important relationships, and showed us what we must work on.

All through this period I kept thinking about my own brief regression to the scene after my death as an island princess. Finally I asked Anne Tully Ruderman, a colleague who was trained in past-life therapy, to regress me to that island life and finish the story. She did, and the result was an eye opener to me. A brief summary of that session follows:

The princess was in love with a stranger who had reached her little island as the result of a shipwreck. The population resented him, and he finally learned that they were planning to kill him.

Two powerful inhabitants of the island were vying for leadership, and the princess was in a dangerous position herself. When her lover revealed that he had constructed a little boat on the other side of the island, which he planned to use as soon as it was dark, she decided to go with him. He refused to take her, on the ground that the boat was too frail to carry more than one person.

She walked him through the woods to the boat in the deep of night, and just as he was shoving off in his tiny boat she tried to jump into it. He pushed her off with his hands and paddled away so vigorously that she could not possibly catch up with him.

Totally frustrated, she tried to find her way home through the dark woods. In her grief and confusion she walked and walked until she dropped to the ground and died, realizing that she had not only lost her lover but also had betrayed her people to bloodshed by the power-hungry rivals.

That session made me do a lot of rethinking about my present life and about my habit of running away from dilemmas. One of my early associations was the first dilemma I could recall—having to choose between two fathers and my dream of having to choose among a hundred fathers. This firsthand experience of past-life therapy opened my understanding more than any book—more, even, than what my patients reported to me.

In the early '80s the literature on reincarnation was scarce, and books on hypnotic regression to past lives were even scarcer. But then Edith Fiore's best-selling book *You Have Been Here Before* came into my hands, and I was delighted to find that her thoughts and feelings on this subject were very close to what I had expressed in a book of my own, *Who Were You Before You Were You?*

I was even more delighted to discover that quite a few people were practicing past-life therapy, much as I was, and that there was even an organization of professionals for research and practice in this field, complete with a newsletter and a journal.

I learned about the Association for Past-Life Research and Therapies (APRT) through a "chance" meeting with its executive director, Hazel Denning, who is one of a handful of pioneers in this field.

Hazel expressed a deep interest in my work and my theories. After a half-hour discussion, she invited me to give a talk and run a workshop at the association's forthcoming conference in California. I accepted eagerly.

It was heartening for me to meet so many people who were steeped in spiritual concepts—and practiced what they believed. In those days—the early eighties—past-life therapy (PLT) was considered even further out than hypnotism, which was still regarded as nothing more than an entertainment. Many serious therapists who used hypnosis called it "relaxation" and were timid about publishing their findings.

Today, of course, new books on reincarnation and PLT are coming out by the dozen, and readers of these books are eager to undergo this form of therapy. Hollywood has picked up the message and produced some superb movies introducing reincarnation and a more realistic conception of hypnosis.

My presentation at APRT was well received and immediately introduced me to a whole new set of friends. Shortly afterward I was invited to join the faculty, whose aim it was to teach past-life therapy techniques to other professionals. I accepted with enthusiasm.

This little faculty was traveling around the country to hold small seminars. My first experience was in Manhattan, and it pleased me to see that the techniques I had worked out for myself were accepted by sophisticated professionals. I was really getting into the life I had always wanted.

In the ensuing years I served APRT variously as an instructor, as a board member, and as the editor of APRT's journal.

Even before I went to California for the APRT meeting, I attended a seminar in New York City, run by Lynn Sparrow, an expert in this field. Lynn was then program director of the Association for Research and Enlightenment, Inc., better known as A.R.E. She had developed her own method for accessing past lives.

This charismatic young woman captivated her audience in a very few minutes. Her regression strategy, quite different from mine, struck me as sound and thoroughly researched. And when it came time to test it out with the group, it worked. I was deeply impressed and had a strong desire to exchange thoughts with her.

At the end of the seminar I introduced myself to her. She showed great interest in my work with hypnotic regressions. After we had talked for a few minutes, she invited me to give a lecture and run a workshop at the next national conference of the A.R.E.

Headquartered in Virginia, the A.R.E. is energetically working to perpetuate the insights of Edgar Cayce, who is becoming more and more widely known since his death in 1945. My presentation led not only to a second invitation but also to a contract to write a book about my work, as well as an invitation to contribute articles to A.R.E.'s bimonthly magazine, *Venture Inward.* Since introducing me to this spiritual organization, Lynn Sparrow has become a valued friend and an inspiration.

Both the A.R.E. and APRT, simply by the fact of their existence, have helped to build a conviction within me that whatever happens to me happens for a reason and that I am in control of the way I handle it. This philosophy embraces even my handicap. I feel quite sure now that nothing is pure chance. I am not afraid to make a decision because, if I muff it, I believe I will have another opportunity—in this life or the next.

I like to think that APRT and A.R.E. are fellow travelers in a quest that I have joined.

TO PHYSICIANS AND SURGEONS AND PSYCHO-THERAPISTS: There are certainly more than enough case histories in the archives of medicine to indicate that standard treatments are not the only road to well-being. Unfortunately, most professionals tend to cling to the training they have undergone, especially if that training was excellent. Medical practitioners have been through training that is virtually incomparable, and they have performed miracles of healing with their hard-bought expertise. I can understand how difficult it must be for them to embrace new theories that have not received an official stamp of approval. But they do eventually open their minds to new ways.

Hypnosis, which doctors generally rated on a level with parlor games, has been winning wide acceptance as a therapeutic tool in very recent years. Past-life therapy is beginning to find its way into medicine's arsenal. Best of all, I find that doctors, like so many others, are beginning to look inward for a deeper meaning in these troubled times.

Whether you take my past-life regression literally or metaphorically, it has done wonders to help me understand my almost lifelong habit of running away from dilemmas. This new understanding put me to work on dealing with this trait. Being presented with choices is no longer a harrowing experience for me. I have come to love choices as opportunities to take charge of my life. If I have the power to choose, I am no longer handicapped in the deepest sense. I know now that being able-minded is more important than being able-bodied.

CHAPTER
25

" . . . AND DON'T FORGET TO DANCE!"

Why do I bring transsexualism into the story of my quest? Let me try to explain. In my groping for a meaning to this strange phenomenon I came on a case that enlarged my understanding of the words "masculine" and "feminine" and my faith in the power that lies within us all.

Nobody really knows why, from time immemorial, certain individuals are convinced that they were born into bodies of the wrong sex and have no peace until this biological anomaly is corrected. The medical profession, led by Harry Benjamin, has found ways to change the body's sexual characteristics and bring peace to these unhappy people.

The program, which takes at least two years, consists of intensive psychotherapy, hormone treatments, and finally surgery. My role in this program is to evaluate the validity of a sex-change candidate's needs and, when appropriate, refer him (or her) on to an endocrinologist and a surgeon.

I had been doing this as a subspecialty for some years when a deeply spiritual but confused transsexual was referred to me to see if I could help him resolve his dilemma. Stan had been in therapy for gender disorder in his hometown, but came to me for a weekend of intensive work. He had a feeling that he might find some deep spiritual answers by letting me regress him to a previous lifetime. His history disclosed all the well-known signs of transsexualism.

After some twenty years of marriage, Stan's dilemma was a conflict between his need to undergo a sex change and his desire to be a good husband to his beloved wife and a good father to his four beautiful children, whom he loved dearly.

Stan's wife was willing to put up with his cross-dressing—that is, wearing clothes of the opposite sex—which he indulged in privately, but both of them knew that a sexchange would destroy their family life.

In our first three sessions, Stan regressed to the same past life as a woman named Laurice, who lived in an old European village. There were many scenes, but what they added up to was a passionate love affair in which Laurice and her lover—later her husband—were constantly dancing together.

Laurice's joyful love life lasted a good fourteen years, but one day it was tragically cut short by a bullet from an unknown source. After a mystical death experience, Laurice found herself in the body of a male infant, angry and lonely, because somehow she knew it was the wrong body.

As he grew up in this current life, Stan made friends with a high-school classmate named Monica. Coming out of hypnosis in my office, he realized that Monica was the same person as the man Laurice had loved so much in that previous lifetime.

At our last hypnotic session, Stan found himself in a woods. "I am Laurice in Stan's body," he said.

And then he saw a goddess in blue, who told him, "You have much to teach yourself as Stan. And you have much to teach others as well. You can always be the woman you want to be, but in Stan's body. So take great care of that body—and don't forget to dance!"

"I can do it," Stan told me. And when I asked him to envision himself as he might be in the future, he saw himself at work with a social service group, doing public speaking and writing—all with the message to his fellow human beings that men as well as women can call on "the eternal feminine" within themselves to find beauty and joy and spiritual fulfillment.

In another snapshot of the future, Stan pictured a visit from Monica, his high-school friend. Monica and her husband were having dinner with Stan and his wife, and they all seemed to be connected by a deep current of warmth and understanding. Stan summed it up with these words: "I've got it all."

———

TO THE HANDICAPPED: I have brought Stan's case into my narrative because I feel that it has a strong healing implication for myself—though I have no gender problem—and therefore, perhaps, for many other handicapped individuals. I, too, have felt trapped in the wrong body. Stan was born into his, but I acquired mine when polio struck me at the age of fourteen months. His physical condition is curable. Mine is not.

Stan chose to reject the transformation of his body, which he had always dreamed of. Two years after his decision he visited me again, but not for a gender problem. He reported that he is living contentedly with his "wrong body." It took me many years before I could say the same about myself.

If you regard your handicap as something more than an inconvenience, I would suggest that you take a deep look inward, possibly using meditation or self-hypnosis, or getting the help of a sympathetic professional. Ask yourself whether your handicap has put you in touch with a spiritual part of yourself.

If your handicap is a lifelong condition, and you have no interest in making that contact inwardly, I would suggest that you devote all your energies to material achievements. That way you will build up your own ego strength. Obviously the spiritual path is not for you—at least not at this point.

I certainly do not want to belittle material achievements. They are important. But if you have made that contact with your Creator, you have found something far more precious than conventional success, and you will be well on your way to inner peace. You will also attract kindred spirits who are eager to make the kind of discoveries you have made.

Most of all, you will recognize that your handicap is a wonderful opportunity to bring meaning and certainty into your life.

TO DOCTORS AND THERAPISTS: Stan's case, while it deals particularly with a gender problem, seems to open the way for new thinking on many other kinds of patients who seek medical help. It suggests that at least for some handicapped persons medication and surgery are not the only routes to healing. Perhaps the day is not too far off when more doctors and therapists will recognize that spiritual guidance can be equally valuable, or, as in Stan's case, far more so.

I would suggest that when a handicapped patient seeks

your help, the anamnesis should include some sympathetic probing into his attitudes and his relationships. If you discover a poor self-image or low self-esteem related to his handicap, it may be that dealing with those symptoms is as important as medicine and surgery in improving the quality of your patient's life.

CHAPTER
26

WHAT ABOUT KARMA?

As my interest in metaphysics expanded, I came increasingly to the belief that whatever happens, happens for a reason—a reason established by whatever Higher Power is looking after us. As a therapist, I saw more and more evidence that some of these reasons go back to previous lifetimes. So I couldn't help wondering if my polio was caused by something that happened long before I was born into my present life.

In all the eleven years during which I underwent conventional psychoanalysis, my polio came in for only the most casual kind of mention. I'm afraid I was trying to pretend to myself (and my analyst) that it was really a very unimportant factor—and I was somehow able to steer both of us away from the topic. But the question never stopped nagging me: Was my polio pure happenstance, or was it bestowed on me for a reason?

It was many years before I worked up the courage to explore that question. At long last I asked Tully, who was not only a capable hypnotherapist but a valued friend as well, to help me find an answer. Tully put me into a trance, and I regressed to a lifetime that had nothing to do with the question I had posed. Figuring that I might be ducking the question, I made another appointment.

On the way home I began to get some feeling of why I didn't want to find the answer I was seeking. Perhaps the answer was something shameful or frightening, and I was showing the well-known phenomenon of resistance.

Before our next session, however, my inner mind must have braced me to deal with it. Tully took me all the way back to ancient Greece, where I was apparently a man of means, occupying an official position of some importance in my city. I had an attractive wife and a charming little girl, whom I loved with a special tenderness.

When Daphne, my daughter in that life, was seven or eight years old she became friendly with a little boy who lived next door. Neleus, as this child was named, walked with a severe limp because one of his legs had been shrunk by disease. He was a likable boy, and I had no qualms about letting my daughter play with him—even after their friendship had gone on for four or five years and it was becoming clear that Daphne was getting more and more attached to him.

The boy's limp was becoming more conspicuous as his body grew up faster than his stricken leg, but this in no way seemed to dampen Daphne's affection for him. I reasoned, however, that my daughter would soon be interested in young men with strong, athletic bodies, and I didn't let myself worry about her "strange friendship" (as I thought of it) until she was seventeen years old. At about that time we had a scene, which I relived vividly in my hypnotic regression.

We were in my home, and Daphne, her eyes shining, was showering me with the news that Neleus this day had proposed to her—and that she had accepted. My reaction was one of shock and outrage.

I told my daughter immediately and in strong language that under no circumstances was this marriage going to take place—no child of mine was going to be married to a cripple! She must get that idea out of her head right now and forever.

"Why, Father? Why?" Daphne pleaded tearfully. "Neleus is a wonderful man!"

I tried to calm down so that I might express my views to her in a more restrained manner. "No cripple can be a wonderful man," I explained gently. "They are all alike—cowardly, dependent, sponging on others, useless appendages on the body of society. You could never be happy with such a person, Daphne."

"But Father, Neleus is not like that. He's the most wonderful young man I know."

I felt my anger surfacing again. "Daphne," I told her quietly, "I have said all I am going to say on this matter. There will be no marriage between you and Neleus. That is all."

That night Daphne stabbed herself to death.

In the next scene of my regression my wife was telling me with great bitterness in her voice, "You killed our daughter! You did it just as surely as if you had plunged that knife into her breast yourself."

I found myself arguing that I was only trying to do what was right in the interest of our daughter's future happiness. But my arguments seemed to make no impression on my wife—or, for that matter, on me. Though I kept on trying in the succeeding days to convince myself that I was blameless in this tragedy, I could apparently do nothing to allay my feelings of guilt and grief. Those feelings followed me to the very end of that life—and into my present life. The session with Tully certainly answers my question about the reason for my handicap.

There is a beautiful postscript to this story. In one of my talks at an A.R.E. conference I told the story of my regression to my life as Daphne's father. Next day, at the same conference, I conducted a workshop. As part of it, I did a group hypnosis and asked the hypnotized participants to go back to some previous lifetime.

At the end of the session, a vividly pretty young woman came up to the platform and grasped my hand. "Guess who I am!" she said with an animated twinkle.

I pleaded a terrible memory for connecting names and faces. But she quickly came to my rescue.

"I'm Daphne!"

The name hit me like a bolt of lightning as the ancient guilt jumped up inside me. I soon learned, however, that I was totally forgiven for my destructive arrogance in that distant incarnation and that this delightful young woman actually wanted to be my friend.

We have been corresponding ever since, and I always look forward to her lively letters which begin, "Dear Daddy."

———

TO HANDICAPPED YOUNGSTERS WHO QUESTION THE GODS: Is my polio in this twentieth-century life a punishment for letting my unfeeling attitude bring about my daughter's death two thousand years ago? I don't think so. I don't hold with the eye-for-an-eye school of thought, nor can I imagine a Supreme Being so punitive as to reincarnate us for the sole purpose of making us pay for our misdeeds, transgressions or errors or blind spots in a previous life.

It's true that when I was young, in my present life, I shook my fist at the skies and asked, "Why me?" But more recently—and particularly since my regression to the life of

Daphne's father—the question I ask is, "Am I learning?"

If, like me, you have wanted to shout at the skies in anger, consider what a handicap has done for me—and what it can do for you. It has enlarged my understanding of the afflictions of others. It has broadened my horizons and made me, I hope, a more compassionate human being.

I like to think of each new incarnation as another opportunity to grow, starting pretty much where I left off in a previous life. I certainly don't want to approach my final years with any other kind of belief. I hold to the conviction that every bit of growth I can achieve in this life will help me get off to a better start in the next one. And that makes the challenges of living worth meeting right up to the moment of death.

Let me try to elaborate on how I feel my handicap has worked for me. In my younger days in this life, I had much of the same arrogance I displayed in that Greek incarnation. Though I succeeded in hiding it, I was inwardly disdainful of persons who were—in what I felt was my expert opinion—stupid, mercenary, meek, overbearing, pretentious, dull, or what have you. In short, the arrogance and shortsightedness I exhibited in my Greek life seemed to cling to me in this one.

Underneath this arrogance, of course, was a deep sense of my own inadequacy—rarely, if ever, consciously acknowledged. After all, anybody could see that I was just like Neleus. I was unable to compete with the able-bodied in strength, in speed, in grace, in sporting skills—in so many of the physical attributes we all admire.

As these bare facts gradually became more and more difficult to deny, my arrogance began to fall away, making room inside of me for feelings of shame, and then for a new humility. The humility, in turn, taught me to understand and then to identify with the very people I formerly would have relegated to the "lower orders," or trolls, including some wonderful handicapped persons.

Finally I came to understand that my disdain for others was really a projection of my own feelings about myself.

One happy result of these new understandings was that casual friends began moving closer to me. I now have ever-deepening relationships with men and women whom I used to keep at a distance out of fear that they would brush me aside.

My new humility also drew me into an intensified inward search that led me, step by step, into the realm of metaphysics and a conviction that I am here for a purpose. If I had grown up with an unimpaired body, I might have set my sights on material success and contented myself with a comfortable life style. I might never have gone into such exciting fields as hypnotism and past-life therapy.

Looking back, I see my handicap as a karmic gift—a gift that has made my life purposeful and meaningful.

So my message to other handicapped individuals is simple: Accept what is given to you, and make the most of it.

CHAPTER
27

DEEP CALLETH UNTO DEEP

Reviewing my years as a psychotherapist, I am surprised to see how much I have learned from my patients. I find that every session is a meeting of inner minds.

One lesson that has profoundly affected the way I see people is the revelation that the world is not divided into the good guys and the bad guys, or the trolls and the nontrolls.

Another lesson is that it is dangerous to judge people. I could go on, but I'd rather give some illustrative cases.

ELMER, a successful businessman, came to me in a state of turmoil and anger because his daughter was going to marry a black man. He had told her that if she went through with this, he would banish her from his house and his heart.

His racism made *me* angry—so angry that I was on the point of telling him to find another therapist. But before I could say anything, a scene from one of my own past-life regressions flashed through my mind—the one cited above in which I was telling my teen-ager in ancient Greece, "No daughter of mine will ever marry a cripple!"

As you know, she killed herself, and my guilt pursued me even into the twentieth century. My polio in this life has given me the chance to atone for my destructive prejudice. I recalled Christ's admonition: "Let him who is without sin cast the first stone." I realized that I still would not be without sin if I cast out a fellow human being who came to me to be healed.

I told Elmer my story. Then I said, "I think I can help you." And I think I did.

ALICIA was one of the first patients to impress me with the enormous power of the inner mind—the unconscious, as Freud and Jung called it. She was suffering from severe migraine headaches, insomnia, and a host of other symptoms. Our first session, I felt, got nowhere. Under hypnosis she produced a series of fragmentary images that seemed to be utterly disconnected.

She came in beaming for her second session. "I don't know what you've done," she said. "I've been feeling just wonderful."

Actually I hadn't done anything, and neither had she. But the explanation for this result hit me like a thunderbolt: Her inner mind had put all those fragments together and endowed them with meaning—a meaning that neither Alicia nor I could consciously understand. But we could both feel it. For Alicia it was healing. For me it was a revelation: You don't always have to know what heals you.

Alicia's experience, which has been matched by many other patients of mine, got me thinking about the Night Visitors I had seen in my childhood—the Little Old Man, the demonic faces, and finally the beautiful Goddess whose very presence was assurance, though I may never know exactly why.

Alicia, though she didn't know it, had given me the key to a new kind of understanding—the understanding of feeling. I have stopped playing the psychoanalytic detective in the landscape of the inner mind, whether it be mine or my patient's. I have learned trust.

In this context I can't refrain from passing along a similar true story that was told to me by a psychiatrist-friend of mine. His wife had a constellation of problems; so he arranged for her to see a colleague—a psychoanalyst with excellent credentials.

Janice, the patient, went four times a week to lie on the couch and say whatever came into her head. She did so for session after session, but after a few months she noticed that her analyst was more and more given to silence. Finally he stopped speaking altogether. He would just sit back and let her do all the talking. Then there came a day when the good doctor was taken away to a mental hospital. But Janice? She was doing just fine—she was cured!

RORY, another patient, was a dynamic extrovert who worshiped the great god Mammon. As a tax consultant to the rich and famous, he was earning an average of $300,000 a year, he told me, but he and his beautiful wife were spending $325,000 a year to maintain their life style. He was desperately trying to boost his income, even though he knew that he would never be satisfied with what he made.

When I asked Rory about his marriage, he said he hardly ever gave it any thought. It didn't matter to him whether he was married or not, though he had nothing to say against his wife. He was too busy trying to jack up their income to give her much thought.

"Money is power," he said many times. "It's the rich who run the country." And with his insider knowledge of the wealthy and the mighty, he had many stories of greed and corruption to support his views.

My own feeling is that the pursuit of money can become

an obsession that takes much of the joy out of life. We had many lively discussions about that.

After a few months, Rory's eloquence was beginning to make me question my own deepest convictions. And when he broke off his therapy without explanation, I wondered whether my defense of my belief that there are more important things in life than money was just the rationalization of a man who would never get rich.

Come Christmas, my wife and I received a giant basket of poinsettias from Rory and his wife. When I called their home to thank them, it was Edith who answered. "Garrett," she exclaimed, "you have no idea what Rory's sessions with you have done for us! He's a new man!"

Rory got on the phone and elaborated. He said the sessions had made him reexamine his values, especially his feelings about Edith. They were both in love all over again, he reported.

I had to do a lot of reexamining of my own feelings about money. As a child, Daddy O.'s hand-to-mouth life style had virtually convinced me that the pursuit of money was an ignoble interference with the spiritual quest.

It is not. Man does not live by bread alone. But neither does he live by love alone. He cannot for long engage in the spiritual quest on an empty stomach. Nor can he deny the needs of the wonderful body his Creator gave him. The body's needs are modest. The spirit's needs are enormous.

———————

TO PSYCHOTHERAPISTS: Helping unhappy or confused, derailed people to turn their lives around is one of the most fulfilling occupations I can think of. But what I didn't realize when I was still dreaming of becoming a psychotherapist was that this kind of help is a two-way street.

All of us, of course, are always learning as we go through life, whether from teachers and books, or from our own mistakes, or from our interchanges with other people—family, friends, children, and business associates. But rarely in all these contacts do people open up and reveal their innermost selves—their core personalities.

We all have what you might call mask personalities to present in the different situations we encounter. We have one personality to display in our work environment, another when we are making love, and still another when we are making a purchase, and so on.

In the psychotherapist's office, however, it's a different story. This is where people come to reveal their innermost emotions, their secret hopes and fears, their loves and hates, their spiritual experiences, their most beautiful dreams and their nightmares—even the secrets they may keep from their friends and their spouses.

The psychotherapist who can offer empathy and establish trust can communicate with this core personality. My own history has enabled me to tell patients in all sincerity that I can understand their problems. Very often I can tell them that I've been through the same thing myself and show them what I've learned in the way of help. My own experiences have made me sensitive to their deepest needs. In return, their confidences have steadily deepened my own exploration of the world beyond the visible.

CHAPTER
28

EIGHTEEN MONTHS TO LIVE

I've been a "terminal" patient for well over ten years now, and these have been the best years of my life.

It all started with a couple of strange yellow streaks that gradually developed on my forearms. I took little notice of them at first, assuming that I had spilled some stain or chemical on my skin and that the streaks—or striae, as the doctors call them—would presently go away. Instead, they developed into broad bands, running from close to the palm all the way up to the crook of the elbow on each arm.

After a few months I showed them to my family doctor, who questioned me closely on my diet and on any skin or hair products I might have used. He finally guessed that the culprit might be the conditioner I was using on my hair. So I wrote a letter to the manufacturer, asking if they had any data on this phenomenon. They didn't. In fact, they were just as puzzled as I was.

After months of resisting my doctor's suggestion that I see a dermatologist, I finally made an appointment with Dr. Jim Baral. This specialist, another careful man, told me not to worry, that the streaks were probably insignificant. But just to be sure, he sliced off a couple of samples of my skin to have them lab-tested.

Two weeks later he informed me of the result: I had multiple myeloma, an incurable form of cancer. He broke the news to me gently enough, but of course it came as a crusher. I immediately thought of the loved ones I would be leaving, of all the unfinished projects I was engaged in, all the old scores I had to settle, all the fences I wanted to mend, and the many modest ambitions I hoped to fulfill. But I was too confused and angry even to ask the usual questions, which I'm sure the good doctor was ready to answer.

As I was juggling these thoughts in my mind, I vaguely heard Dr. Baral say that he had never seen striae like mine in such an unusual part of the body as the forearms, and he asked me if I would mind going on exhibition before his colleagues in the medical profession. There were only two similar cases on record, he said. But I was too immersed in my own emotions to give him an answer on the spot, so he urged me to think it over.

When I got home, the first thing I did—after breaking the news to my wife and offering her what inadequate comfort I could—was to pull out my obsolete edition of the *Merck Manual*, the doctor's bible of diseases. I read: "No cure has yet been found for myeloma; death always occurs ... A fatal termination usually may be expected within eighteen months." Many weeks later a subsequent edition of *Merck* gave me this slightly less gloomy outlook: "The median for responding [to some new chemotherapy] patients is two to three years."

Taking eighteen months as my "deadline," I sat down to ponder my meager future. I talked myself into accepting the fact that I'd never get around to writing the book I had in mind. I'd never complete the courses I felt I needed for a future I was never to have. I'd never get to a whole list of other major projects.

But there were some things I still could do. For one thing, I could get in touch with my daughter Lyn in California. Somehow we had drifted apart over the past several years, and I knew I loved her far too much to leave this life without trying to reanimate the beautiful relationship we'd once had. I wrote her a letter to that effect and was rewarded a few days later with a warm phone call. We were soon as beautifully close as we had been in the past.

Since I was in no pain and outwardly symptom-free, except for those yellow streaks, I decided to go on living and learning to the best of my ability—keeping up with friends, continuing to see patients, enjoying my leisure hours, conducting and attending my usual quota of workshops, seminars, and conferences, and generally maintaining my old pace.

All this time, of course, I'd been thinking over Dr. Baral's request that I put myself on exhibition. I didn't like the idea one bit, but I concluded that if in my terminal days I could help to make some small contribution to medical knowledge, it was something I should do.

Two weeks after learning my diagnosis, I went on exhibition at Mount Sinai Medical Center in New York. And shortly after that, I was put on display at the venerable New York Academy of Medicine.

If you've ever felt like a sad, sick fish in a fishbowl, you can begin to appreciate my emotions at these learned gatherings. I had to sit passively and publicly, naked from the waist up, while doctor after doctor came over to me, bent my neck one way or the other, or held up one of my streaked arms, and then the other for closer inspection. Some of the doctors, especially the women practitioners, had a warm greeting for me, but many of the surgeons just manipulated me as if I were a curious specimen and not a person. I remember feeling grateful that none of these frosty specialists had charge of my case.

Two days later I visited Dr. Joseph Glass, a highly respected New York oncologist, to whom I was referred by Dr. Baral. Dr. Glass confirmed that I did indeed have multiple myeloma. The news had no shock value at this point, as I had already accommodated myself to that fact. I did not discuss the prognosis with Dr. Glass, nor did I ask him any questions about my probable longevity—or shortgevity. I was beginning to make my own decisions about that.

A month or so later I attended a meeting of the New York Milton H. Erickson Society for Psychotherapy and Hypnosis (NYSEPH). The speaker was Anne Tully Ruderman, a Westchester psychotherapist who had studied with the well-known oncologist O. Carl Simonton, director of the Cancer Counseling and Research Center in Pacific Palisades, California. I have already mentioned her, but at this point in my life I had not yet met her.

Tully, as I soon came to know her, talked about the Simonton method of instilling a joyful outlook and positive expectations in his patients to reinforce his medical treatment. She told us about his remarkable successes in curing "hopeless cases" of cancer in many patients, extending the life of many others and dramatically improving the quality of life in nearly all.

I was so impressed with both the lecture and the lecturer that I introduced myself to Tully after the program. On learning that her office was just five minutes away from mine (coincidence? tell me!), I asked her if she would take me on as a patient. She said she'd be happy to.

At my first session with her, I was completely delighted by her warmth, her concern, her directness, and her expertise. There was no trace of professional stuffiness about her, and our rapport was almost instant. It increased as the months went by.

Between Dr. Glass's skilled medication for my body and Tully's gentle but deft therapy for my psyche, the spread of my cancer seemed to be slowed down—and then halted. In fact, unless it was an illusion, I felt it was beginning to reverse.

What was the magic of these sessions with Tully Ruderman? Actually we talked very little about my cancer. The focus was rather on my attitudes and on the many personal difficulties in my life. Little by little I found myself dealing with those attitudes and problems in new ways.

Most notably, perhaps, I was much more relaxed. I no longer felt under enormous pressure to achieve the goals I had set for myself before learning my prognosis. Instead, I was learning to enjoy the process of *working toward* those goals—and the likelihood of that process being interrupted by an early death was beginning to lose its terrors.

The imminence of death was in fact making me take a new look at the world around me. And everything in that world began to look more precious than it had ever seemed before; every moment more pregnant with meaning. Without consciously trying, I found myself squeezing the essence out of each daily experience, making the most of every little bit of time that was left to me. This was soon to become my way of life.

On the medical front, meanwhile, my lab tests were consistently showing a downward trend in my protein level. The day came when the doctor informed me that the level had dropped to normal and there was no trace left of the cancer. "You can discontinue all medication," he said. It's been that way ever since.

On the professional front, I was definitely upgrading my skills as a therapist. Today I no longer torture myself with anxieties about my degree of success or failure with my patients. I know I'm giving them the best I've ever had to offer, and from there on it's up to them. Sensing *my* relaxation, my patients become more confident and gain ground more rapidly in their journey toward wholeness. As a result, my rate of therapeutic success has gone up significantly.

One patient expressed it this way to me after a particularly productive session: "There's some quality in your voice or your manner or something that just makes me feel sure you can help me. You seem to understand."

On the creative front, I've become more productive than ever, writing papers and articles, giving lectures, conducting workshops, and even working on that book I thought I'd never get around to. I was eager to communicate to others whatever insights I had gleaned from my own experiences. The book is now out, and I am getting the kind of feedback from readers that makes me feel my life has been worthwhile—even if it is terminated tomorrow.

On the personal front, the prospect of early death has made me want to leave a little something of myself to each of the people I live with or work with. As a consequence, I think, I've become a more outgoing person. People seem to relate to me in a new, closer way, and this has helped me to like myself a lot better.

On the domestic front, I've discovered so much marital and family happiness that for a long time I felt sure something awful must be about to happen. But nothing awful has happened, and my fear has gradually dwindled to nothing.

In short, my life has never been so good as it is today. Why?

I think the prospect of an early death forced me to take a new look at life and made me realize something I'd often heard but never before appreciated at a gut level—that the length of life is of minor importance compared with its quality.

TO THE HANDICAPPED PERSON FACING DEATH:
Even if you have made peace with your handicap, the news
that you now have a fatal illness on top of it may make you
want to throw up your hands and cry, "Enough, O Lord!
Haven't I paid my dues?" That reaction is perfectly natural,
but it won't do a darned bit of good for you.

Instead of shaking your fist at your Creator, I suggest that
you start asking yourself some important questions, such
as:

Is your present life, as it stands, giving you a sense of fulfillment? Are you giving everything you should to your
marriage (or whatever is your most significant relationship)? Do you maintain a relaxed attitude under the
deadlines and other pressures on your job? Are you and
your loved ones having enough fun? Are you ready to give
up some of your ambitions?

If your answer to these questions, and possibly others, is
No, I would suggest that you do some overhauling—with or
without the help of a psychotherapist, a tax consultant, a
minister or rabbi, or anyone else you can trust.

How do you feel about the prospect of death? Cheated or
content?

And what do you believe happens to your soul after you
cross over? Are you afraid of Hell? Or of ceasing to exist altogether? Or do you think you'll be back on earth in the future
to give it another try?

These are questions that many of us try not to think
about, but this is the very time to face them. Instead of worrying about how many weeks you have left, try cleaning up
your inner household. Realize that your inner life is far more
significant than your earnings. Try mending your relationships. If you take it for granted that you love your wife, tell
her how much you do. Turn your days into fun. And *stop
worrying!*

Easier said than done, you may think. But this is really the time you can put your worries aside and relax. When you can do that, you may prolong your life and even reverse the progress of your illness.

But if these prove to be the last days of your life, by all means do everything you can to make each day wonderful!

CHAPTER
29

IT ALL COMES TOGETHER

If you share my belief that synchronicity is a phenomenon you can count on, you will understand this most
important sequence in my life. By this time, Fae and I were
growing in different directions, and, by friendly agreement,
we were in the midst of preparations for a divorce. It was the
second time we decided to split.

Five or six years earlier, we had retained a divorce lawyer,
but he unexpectedly died before all the details had been
completed, and the divorce did not become final. After that
we decided we'd give our marriage another try. It didn't
work. We were finally convinced that divorce was the only
way to get our individual lives back on track.

At the same time, I was getting deeper and deeper into
my metaphysical quest, trying to find my own personal answers to life's mysteries. That quest led me to a meeting, as I
have said, with Lynn Sparrow and her invitation to speak at

an A.R.E. conference. This, in turn, led to an invitation from a publisher to write a book about my work (which I did) and to another invitation to attend the A.R.E. New Year's conference. It was at this conference that I met Gwen.

Synchronicity? I would say—oh well, let Gwen tell the story in her own words:

"I was looking desperately for some naturopathic cure for a skin condition that had been torturing me for more than twenty years. The medical profession was letting me down miserably, even to the point where I was put on dangerous drugs and feeling suicidal.

"In reading one of Ruth Montgomery's spiritual books, I noticed the name and address of the A.R.E. in Virginia Beach, Virginia. I quickly applied for membership and received some literature on healing with the mind.

"I was especially impressed by some books about Edgar Cayce which described his techniques for healing psoriasis and other skin conditions. I read them eagerly, thinking that maybe there was some hope for me.

"Not long afterward I received a brochure in the mail describing the A.R.E.'s forthcoming New Year's conference. I began to feel that I was being pointed in a new direction, and I promptly made arrangements to attend.

"I was looking for answers to some important questions that were on my mind: Why do I have this condition? What have I done to bring it onto me? What do I need to learn in order to solve this problem once and for all? Or, conversely, how can I live with it in peace?

"Much of my reading had already convinced me that reincarnation is a fact. It was as if a light had gone on inside of me—I just knew it was true. The idea that people have had past lives and can expect to have future lives just made sense to me. I was unaware at the time that past-life regressions were beginning to be an accepted mode of therapy.

"One of my many dermatologists had told me emphatically that I must change my way of life completely. I told him that this was impossible. But a week after that I had a change of heart; I checked into moving to Arizona, the state with a perfect climate for people with allergies.

"I couldn't bring myself to make the move. Leaving my family, my job, my friends, my roots was simply out of the question. However, the thought kept bugging me: A change in my life was a must if I wanted to survive.

"At the conference, I was drawn into a conversation with a man who was sitting in the row just ahead of me and a little to my right. We were waiting for the conference to begin. Morris Netherton, a pioneer in past-life therapy, was the featured speaker.

"In the course of our discussions, I learned that my new friend was a past-life therapist himself. I was enthralled. During a recess I got up the courage to ask him if there was a chance he might help me with my physical problem. We arranged to have weekly sessions at his office in Tappan, New York.

"In a very short time the relief I experienced was nothing short of dramatic. But soon, in the course of my therapy, I began to feel more strongly that the dermatologist was right when he said I must change my way of life completely. Moving away from home would mean letting go of some relationships that had meant a lot to me. Would I really be strong enough to do it? I wasn't at all sure of that. What I was altogether sure of now was that it needed to be done. Like it or not, I must do it.

"During my weekend sessions in New York, Garrett's wife Fae and I soon became friends. I could see that her marriage to Garrett was in troubled waters. When I learned that a divorce was imminent and that Garrett was going to need help in his work, I struck a deal with him: I would help run the business end of his practice as well as his household in exchange for a small salary plus room and board.

"This was agreeable to all of us and would give me the opportunity to start my new life. Back home I had a hard time explaining things to the people I loved, but they all said they would support the move if it meant a happier life for me.

"During the difficult year that followed, my relationship with Garrett grew more and more intense. One day he told me that he loved me. I told him that I loved him, too, and it was not long afterward that we were married."

My marriage to Gwen is something special. It was wonderful to discover that she was a person I couldn't fight with—this in spite of the fact that we work together all day and stay together through the evening and the night. We can argue. We can sometimes see things differently. At times we can hurt each other's feelings without meaning to. But we just never seem to lose our temper with each other or get into the kind of steamy battles my patients and my friends often talk about. I have still to come upon another couple more attuned to each other than we are.

We have been through some trying times and some tragic times together, including illnesses, deaths, and family problems. But these have always drawn us closer together, because there is always that wonderful underpinning of happiness that keeps us going—the happiness that we have each other.

What brought us together? Coincidence?

———

TO THE HANDICAPPED: Gwen and I firmly believe that we knew each other in a whole string of past lives. A couple of regressions by each of us helped to confirm this in our own minds, though we would never tell anyone else that this is more than impressive evidence.

My union with Gwen has given me a beautiful answer to all the questions that plagued me for so many years—questions about my ability to survive without my mother, questions about my competence to compete for employment in the world of the able-bodied, questions about my attractiveness—or lack of it—to the opposite sex, and on and on.

All these questions can be answered in one word: "Trust." And that is the word I would like to pass on to all handicapped people who may feel cheated on the quality of their life. Trust that whatever is handed to you, including your handicap, is for a reason.

If you rage against life, you will find that it rages right back at you. If you grasp life and take it to your heart with all the joys and challenges it hands you, you will discover that you can be strong and loving and filled with the fun of just being alive.

CHAPTER
30

WHAT'S IN A NAME?

My experiences with the Night Visitors—the Little Old Man, the demons, and the beautiful Goddess—combined to build up my conviction that the visible world around me is not the only reality.

I wanted passionately to restore the sense of connection with the great Creative Force that I knew was out there. But it was a quest I kept on hold for long periods in order to take care of pressing mundane problems—problems like earning a living and parenting a lively child.

Whenever I saw a chance, however, I tried to pursue my vision—alone or with the help of gifted people. I've consulted astrologers, psychics, channels, dowsers, tarot card readers, scryers, even a man who uses a computer to read the stars.

The results have ranged all the way from revelations to disappointments. The reason for this mixture, of course, lies

in the fact that in the metaphysical world not all practitioners are equally gifted. There are the amazingly gifted,
the less gifted, and the not gifted. I would rank computers
among the not-at-all gifted.

Not long ago Gwen and I had computerized astrology
readings. Among the many findings, I was told that I had
married Gwen for her wealth and her connections to important people. The truth is that when Gwen came to me
she was in very modest circumstances and had no idea of
who those "important people" might be.

Gwen's reading took place at the same time with the same
person. She was told that she had married me for my money
and my connections to important people. Actually my only
wealth was the modest house I lived in, on which I owed a
considerable mortgage loan, and my acquaintance with
important people was a now-and-then kind of pleasure. I
could have told that astrologer exactly why we married. It
was purely and simply for love.

Now let me give you an example of mixed results. During
my previous marriage I learned about a little town in Florida
called Cassadaga. It was really more of a community than a
town, and its inhabitants were psychics. They called themselves mediums in those days, and they had won such a
reputation for accurate readings that Hollywood stars
would regularly make special trips across the continent to
consult them.

Fae and I were planning to visit her brother Bert, who
lived in Florida, and we decided to stop at Cassadaga. I
made an early morning appointment with one of the
community's most prominent mediums.

The community consisted of tiny cottages that circled a
lake. On our arrival it was veiled in a soft mist that gave it a
storybook atmosphere.

We spent the night before our appointment at
Cassadaga's only hotel, which also served as the town's

shopping center. It was a pleasantly run-down building, and we sat for a few hours in the social room, being very careful not to let out any information about ourselves.

Next morning, at eight o'clock sharp, we drove up to our medium's cottage. She was a gray-haired, pleasant-looking woman who was busy tending the flowers in her front yard. After we introduced ourselves, we were invited to go inside. As we were walking in, she turned to me and said, "I'll tell you something: Your father carried a cane, just like you do, only he didn't need it."

That was a hit. My father did indeed carry a cane, but only because he liked to. I carried a cane to help me walk. The hit diluted my skepticism by at least fifty percent and got us off to a running start. We went into the cottage and made ourselves comfortable. But from there on, it was a hit-and-miss experience.

Another example of a hit: "I'm getting the name Bert—or is it Bertie?" Turning to Fae, she said, "He must be somebody very important to you."

"He's my brother," Fae acknowledged. She explained that her mother had named him Bertie, but when he grew up he was better known as Bert.

An example of a miss by a mile: Turning to me, this nice lady said firmly: "Your future is in Florida."

I have never been back to Florida since that time, which was many years ago. But sometimes I wonder: Did I miss my future?

The rest of the session went on like that for about an hour. At the end the medium charged us $5. It was well worth it.

Years later, when Gwen and I were married, I asked her "How do you feel about psychics?"

She said, "Let me tell you about some experiences I had before I ever knew you." It turned out that her feelings were much the same as mine, although she had consulted just two psychics in her life. "The second one was a total washout. The first—well . . . "

I pressed her for details, and got this story:

"About six months before you and I met at the A.R.E., one of my best friends urged me to see Gloria, a psychic she knew very well. 'It can't hurt,' she argued, and I had to agree. After all, my doctors weren't doing all that great. To them, my future looked pretty bleak, medically speaking. They told me there was no cure for my problem; I just had to learn to live with it.

"My own feeling was that I had a better prospect than they would allow. I was learning that doctors don't know it all. So I phoned Gloria for an appointment.

"Her office was in a small, sort of mall-like setting. I had guessed that she would look like a gypsy and would have a picture of Jesus on the wall. I was right about the picture of Jesus, but Gloria didn't look the least bit like a carnival figure. She was a light-skinned, black-Oriental woman. There was something mystical about her, but her manner was gracious and sincere. I liked her immediately.

"In her office, Gloria explained how she worked. She would go into a light trance while her special spirit connection gave her images that would be pertinent to me and my questions. After a few moments of silence she began speaking again. I enjoyed my interaction with her very much, but didn't feel that a psychic connection had truly occurred.

"She told me that the middle finger on my right hand would be severely injured and that I might lose it if I wasn't careful."

I asked Gwen, "Did you injure it?"

"Yes. I was opening a can of vegetables and cut my finger rather badly, but it didn't require any stitches. It was the middle finger, all right. But that could have been just a coincidence.

"After Gloria warned me about my finger, she made a lot

of other predictions that sounded questionable to me. I began to feel that I had wasted $40, even though I enjoyed my connection with her.

"About halfway through our session, she asked me to turn off my tape recorder. She had some very private and special information to relay to me from her source.

"Then she said, 'You will become involved with a man. He has a mustache. He walks with a limp. There's something at his side—I can't make it out. The initials of his first name are J.J.—I believe it's James or Joseph. No, it's James Joseph. Do you know someone by that name?'

"I told her, 'No. I really have no desire to become involved with anyone.'

"But she went right on: 'This man will become very close. You will work together, or maybe you are working together now. Do you know anyone who fits this description?'

"I shook my head and insisted that it could not and would not be. There was just no interest. At this we concluded our session and had a very nice chat."

After Gwen finished her story, we both remained silent for long minutes. I saw that Gwen was looking at me intently.

"Good grief!" she suddenly exclaimed. "You fit the picture! You have a mustache. You walk with a limp. That thing she said was at your side, that's your cane! And we work together, and we've become involved, just like she said."

Gwen looked totally amazed for a moment. Then her expression changed. "But how about that name she gave me? I don't see how you can get James Joseph out of Garrett— not if you tried all night.

"Hey! Garrett! What's the matter?"

I was stunned. Only now did I realize that I had been listening for some time with my mouth wide open. As soon as I could pull myself together, I said, "Listen to this, Gwen. I'll start at the beginning.

Before my brother Ralph was born, I told Gwen, his paternal grandmother wanted him to be named Joseph in memory of her deceased husband. My Daddy O. didn't like that name, so he stuck with the name Ralph. Grandma O. and a lot of other relatives thought that wasn't nice of him.

When I came along, however, the pressure was stepped up, and my dad finally decided on a compromise. I would be named James after my father. Who could argue with that? But I would have Joseph as my middle name, which I could abbreviate to an initial. So my name came out James J. Oppenheim.

Now it was Gwen's turn to listen with an open mouth. We both agreed that this was too much to explain by coincidence. Keep in mind that Gwen had never met me when she visited Gloria. She hadn't even heard of me at all. And neither had Gloria.

"So how did James Joseph get to be Garrett then?" Gwen asked. And I told her the rest of the story.

When I started to send out my immature poems under the name James J. Oppenheim, it was soon obvious that the editors thought they were my father's, and that his work had radically deteriorated. I began to feel that I was doing Daddy O. a serious disservice—that my poems were just another negative reflection of him. I really wanted an identity of my own.

So I began submitting my work under the name J.J. Oppenheim. I thought I had found a solution until one of my poems came back from the *American Mercury*, a prestigious literary magazine, with a personal note from H.L. Mencken, its eminent editor. The note read: "Jimmy, I wish you'd turn to prose!"

That did it. I told my father I must change my name—for his sake, I added. On one of my visits to him, we all sat around for a full evening trying out names on one another. None of them seemed to sit right with me.

Somehow the conversation turned to poetry and the hard lot of poets, who usually go unappreciated and starve in a garret.

Garret! I liked the sound of it. I thought it went nicely with my last name. It also seemed to define me as a person and a poet in my own right—not just a reflection of my father. We all agreed that it made a good name, and I added an extra *t* to the end of it to give it some solidity.

My relatives and friends had a hard time accepting it. They treated me as though God had given me the name James, and I had no right to change it. "It was good enough for your father," some of them pointed out. But I insisted that I was now Garrett and would they please get used to that.

The name had a profound emotional effect on me. I was no longer James Junior. I was me!

My mother, of course, was the last holdout. In fact, she didn't come around until I was married to Dona, who added her insistence to mine. Looking back on that marriage, this is one of the memories that makes me feel grateful to Dona.

———

TO PARENTS: "That which we call a rose by any other name would smell as sweet." So says the poet. And I am glad that Shakespeare attributed this shaky aphorism to a teen-ager who was in love and not to himself—because "it ain't necessarily true." If you were to call a rose a stinkweed, a lot of people would feel differently about it. And if you were to call a mouse Michelangelo, I think the little creature would have a loving, respectful following.

Names have connotation. Suppose you were writing a novel. Would you call the hero Ichabod? Names have sounds that can please or displease. More than that, they have associations, they stir up images. For me, the name Ichabod brings up the image of Ichabod Crane, the scared and skinny schoolmaster depicted by Washington Irving in *The Legend of Sleepy Hollow.*

Names can inspire family pride. James, for example, brings to mind a succession of English monarchs. For me, as a child, that name was a proud identification with the daddy I idolized. But when I grew up, the name James kept whispering to me that I had no identity of my own.

Parents, when naming a newborn child, have only their own preferences to go by, since the baby has no voice in the matter. And coming to the point of this little essay, I would advise parents to honor their child's desire to change his name if he wants to. And that applies particularly to a handicapped child, who may be deeply troubled about his own identity.

Discuss his wishes, by all means. Encourage him to air his reasons. Some of them, like the wish to have an identity separate from his father's, may be difficult for him to tell you. If you suspect such a reason, bring it up yourself, and then ask him how he feels about it.

CHAPTER
31

HOW TO ATTRACT ENEMIES

You may recall William, the bully I had to contend with in the special class for handicapped children. Looking back, it seems to me that until a few years ago I always had an enemy—someone who could fill me with fear or rage or shame, someone who could plague my nights with anticipations or sap my energy by day.

I don't remember every one of them, and I won't even try to list all that I do remember. I will merely describe some of the outstanding ones, and what I believe this phenomenon has meant to me. Perhaps it has something to do with my karma—the opportunity to cope with my own deficiencies: shame, cowardice, and fantasies of omnipotence.

It may even be that I created my own enmities. As a therapist, I have come to suspect that if a person gets into the same kind of trouble over and over, he must have a hand in bringing it about. Maybe I needed some education in handling these situations.

My stepfather's advice for handling William—"Give him back two for one"— didn't always work for me. Some enemies were much bigger or stronger than I; they would come back four for two, leaving me beaten, shamed, and raging. Or worse, they would simply brush me off, leaving me humiliated and hangdoggy.

The apartment house in which I lived with my parents was separated from the adjoining building by a very narrow courtyard, a sort of alley. My bedroom was on that alley, and a few feet below my window was a window on the other side. The tenant of the room behind that window came home around midnight every night and would then open the window, get out his ukelele, and sing in a loud voice while he strummed:

> Just one more time,
> Just one more time . . .

And so on. For some reason known only to himself, he would repeat this same refrain over and over till about 3 a.m. After the first few nights of this, I felt I couldn't take much more; and neither, apparently, could several of the neighbors. Some of them would shout, "Tone it down! We're trying to get a little sleep!" Some would throw light bulbs that would explode in the courtyard. All this produced no result.

I began shouting across the courtyard myself, but I might as well have been shouting at a phonograph record. I told my parents, and they mentioned it to the superintendent, who promised to talk to the young man. No result. Week after week the disturbance went on until one night, for no reason I could fathom, it stopped.

But all the while it lasted, I would go to bed and wait for the ukulele man to come home and start practicing. "Just one more time, just one more time" got to be a refrain I carried around in my head. It kept reminding me how much feeling of helplessness and anger I was carrying around inside myself.

Years later, when I was appointed chief of the financial copy desk on the *Herald Tribune,* things went fairly well until the arrival of—well, I'll call him Otto. Otto worked on the general news desk and was sent to me on loan when we were shorthanded. He was a lanky, pale, nervous-looking man, and he kept asking me, "How am I doing?"

I gathered that he was struggling with some terrible insecurity, so I would keep telling him, "Don't worry." But I was glad when he went back to general news.

Shortly after that, my desk lost a man. The head of the general news desk promptly offered Otto to fill the gap, and I was urged by management to take him aboard.

On my way out that night, I passed the general news desk. The copy desk chief there, a veteran newsman, swiveled around in his chair to give me a long, long look. There was a foxy twinkle in his eyes, and there was no mistaking the message: "I sure dumped this problem on you!"

Early on, Otto discovered that on certain days we both took the same bus to Rockland County, where my girlfriend Dona was staying with her parents. As we boarded the bus at the George Washington Bridge terminal, I was getting a very bad feeling about Otto. I was a little ahead of him, and I sat down next to someone who had taken a window seat, even though there were other double seats available.

Otto came over and suggested that I move to a seat together with him. I pleaded that I had some reading to do. He was very loud in his insistence, and people were turning their heads; so I moved to a seat on the aisle with Otto, who took the window seat.

He lost no time in asking me, "How am I doing?" I said I didn't want to talk shop right now, but as he kept badgering me, I said, "Don't worry about it. You're doing all right."

I learned later that he quoted my statement at a newspaper guild hearing on his charge against me. Actually, I was having to rewrite practically everything he handled, and I was already keeping major stories away from him.

As the bus rolled on, Otto kept talking in a loud voice about how badly things were going everywhere. "It's the kikes and niggers, lousing everything up," he said in a voice that carried through the bus.

"Excuse me," I said, getting up. "I don't want to hear that kind of talk." And I went to another seat.

Thereafter, it seemed that every time I made any kind of remark to any of the editors on my desk, there would come a loud cackle from Otto, followed by compulsive laughter. He would interrupt me at every possible time and inject comments about the army. He was a veteran of World War I, and I think you may have gathered by now that he was mentally unbalanced. I could forgive his cackles and his snide remarks, but his racism was too much for me.

Presently he lodged a complaint with the newspaper guild's grievance committee on our paper. His major grievance was that I was giving all the big stories to the Jews on my desk. There was a brief hearing at which Otto and I were each called in separately. I gave my opinion that he was irrational, paranoid, and probably in need of professional help. Otto's complaint was dismissed, but he never stopped cackling and laughing his high-pitched, mocking laugh.

I can't say I handled his antagonism too well. I was always torn between my anger over his racism and the feeling that Otto was a very sick man. Whatever happened to him is unknown to me, because I soon switched to a better job on the *New York Times,* and shortly after that the *Herald Tribune* folded up.

Many years later, after Gwen and I were married and I

was absorbing her philosophy of gentleness and under-standing, I got into a different kind of joust.

By accident, in maneuvering my Escort out of a parking place, I grazed the side of a Mercedes that was parked be-hind me, leaving a very small dent. The driver jumped out and started railing at my wife and me. He insisted that we follow him immediately to an auto-body shop he knew.

I said, "I have an appointment in fifteen minutes. Can we make it a little later? You have my license number. I'll meet you there."

He shot back angrily, "*You* inconvenienced *me*. Either you follow me or I'll call the police. And if I do, your insur-ance will go sky-high."

We continued in this vein for another minute or so while I decided that since I had done the damage, I would follow him and be late for my appointment. He was shouting by this time, "Who do you think you are? You think you can go around bumping cars and then just drive off scot-free? This is a $70,000 Mercedes, not (with a contemptuous expres-sion) an Escort!"

I said in a quiet voice, "Calm down. I'll follow you."

He seemed bewildered for a moment or two—like a boxer whose opponent suddenly vanishes. Then he got into his car and led us to a nearby body shop, where he jumped out and had a brief conference with the owner. I'll never know what took place at that conference, but when he came back he said, "You've got to pay for a complete paint job."

He explained angrily that he had just bought the car for $70,000, and that it must be a complete job because other-wise the paint might not exactly match. I must have lifted my eyebrows at that for he immediately added, "If you don't want to, just say so and I'll call the police and your insur-ance will go right up."

Gwen quietly counseled me, "Let's just go along with him so we can get this behind us without hassling." It was as though she was expressing my very own feeling.

The estimate came to more than $1000, and I suggested that we try another body shop for a second estimate. His answer was, "You want me to call the police?"

Gwen again counseled, "It's only money. Why don't you just pay him. Then we can go our way in peace."

I hesitated for a moment because I felt that we were being taken. But then I decided that Gwen was right. It wasn't a battle for money now, even though it was big money; it was a battle of egos. I thought, "Let him gloat over what he's done. I am living a beautiful life with Gwen, and I want to keep it this way. Our peace of mind is worth infinitely more than a thousand dollars."

I wrote a check, and Gwen and I returned to our car. The aggrieved driver came over to us. "I'm sorry I lost my temper," he said. "I see that you are nice people. But that Mercedes is the most precious thing in my life. It's my baby!" He handed me a business card and added, "If you ever need any new furniture, I can give you a good deal."

I accepted his card graciously and gave him mine. "If you ever feel the need for a psychotherapist," I said, "just call my number." And we drove off serenely in our humble Escort.

TO THE HANDICAPPED: We've all observed it: Some people seem to have an absolute genius for getting into the same kind of trouble over and over. Handicapped people more than some others may gave a tendency to fall back on old patterns. Even if those patterns are unhealthy, they have spelled survival. New patterns are scary; one never knows whether he will handle them adequately.

But why do some people manage to get into the same troubles over and over? Psychoanalytic theories provide some plausible explanations, but they don't really explain how an individual can attract or repel other individuals without either of them knowing how it comes about.

As a therapist in search of metaphysical answers, I have come to believe in what lovers call the chemistry of attraction. Many students of metaphysics refer to it as "the law of attraction," one of the universal laws that are said to govern all of us. How we generate that chemistry is still a mystery; but I have come to think of the phenomenon in terms of subliminal body language, popularly known as the "vibes" that we give off. When two strangers are in a room together their bodies are speaking the language of the inner mind, or unconscious if you will. The unconscious messages that our bodies give off are met by the other person's body messages, and right there we may have the beginning of friendship or enmity.

The handicapped person, because of his visible "difference," may have a body language that is more difficult for another person to understand. This can lead to his becoming a target for people who need antagonism in their life.

Understanding this can help you, the handicapped person, to relax with your body so it no longer gives off messages that invite hostile people to take you on.

When you get into a hostile relationship, it helps to think that it was put in your way to help you develop a better sense of your own self-worth.

The above words may look confusing on first reading, but I think that if you study them you may be rewarded with an enhanced ability to form sound relationships.

CHAPTER
32

FAULTS OF THE ANGELS

This chapter is addressed partly to the handicapped, but—more important—to all the people who may cross paths with them in the course of their daily life.

It is hardly surprising that the nicest, kindest, most compassionate people are always ready to lend a hand to a disabled person. But it is not universally realized that there are many situations in which the most willing helper can unwittingly do psychological and even physical harm to the person he wants to help.

What follows is a sampling of my own experiences and whatever wisdom I have extracted from them. I know that some of these experiences will sound unduly trivial, and you may well wonder what this fuss is all about.

But it is precisely these seemingly insignificant instances, which are quickly put aside or passed over, that can wiggle their way into the psyche and damage the individuals they are supposed to help.

If you will give some thought to these examples and, I hope, act on them, I am sure that most of the people who are in the same boat as I am will be as appreciative as I.

THE LUGGAGE-GRABBERS: When Fae left California to marry me, she left many friends and relatives behind. She was delighted when Amy, a special friend, arranged to visit us in New York. At the airport I picked up Amy's suitcase. When she wanted to relieve me of its weight, I insisted on taking it to the car.

Amy was a professional nurse, and I felt she would readily understand my feelings as a handicapped individual; so I took pains to explain them to her on the drive home. It gave me a bad feeling, I told her, whenever I was treated as more disabled than I actually am. Doing whatever I could do not only strengthened my muscles but also made me feel more like a useful member of the human race. Being treated as helpless, however, made me think that this was the way others perceived me.

I told Amy that it delighted me to perform the little courtesies, like opening doors for women or carrying things for them, so long as I could carry them with my one free hand, the other being on my cane. Amy said that she thoroughly understood and that she respected my feelings.

On the night before her departure, Amy packed her suitcase and left it at the front door before we all went to bed. I said I would take it to the car in the morning, and she expressed her thanks.

When I came into the living room in the morning, the suitcase was gone. Fae confirmed that Amy had taken it out in the middle of the night—to spare me.

I confess that I had a hard time restraining myself. All through breakfast and the ride to the airport I was very silent and must have presented a stony appearance. When

Fae and I dropped Amy at the entrance, she turned to me and asked, "What have I done to make you so angry with me?"

I couldn't hold it any longer. I said, "After that talk we had, I thought you understood my feelings. But then you actually went out of your way to show me that you didn't care."

"I'm sorry," was all Amy could muster in reply.

On the way home, I learned that Fae was a party to the suitcase episode. When I expressed my surprise at this, since my wife was thoroughly acquainted with my feelings, she seemed to think that the act was an act of kindness on Amy's part.

I'm sure now that it was, but at the time I was in no mood to believe it. I snapped, "You and your friends could kill me with kindness!"

With the great change in feelings that has come over me in the last five or six years, I have come to regret my behavior. I know that Amy was overriding my objections in order to save me from trouble. If she reads this, I hope she will forgive me.

THE INACCESSIBLES: I was referred to a prominent orthopedist on Park Avenue. When I reached his address, I was surprised to see that there were four or five steps up from the street to his office—and no handrail to hold onto.

After my risky tussle with the stairs, I found that his waiting room was filled with handicapped and elderly patients, several of whom were physically far worse off than I was. I asked this doctor why such an illogical situation had not been corrected simply by installing handrails. He replied that he had long ago requested his landlord to put up a handrail, but so far had not seen any action.

I said, only half in jest, "You can tell your landlord that if I get hurt on those stairs, he's in for one great big beautiful lawsuit."

On my next visit to this orthopedist I found not one, but two solid handrails in place.

If you walk up and down Park Avenue, you will see that most doctors' offices can be reached only by stairs, often without handrails.

I am happy to note a new recognition by our government of the needs of the handicapped for ramps and handrails and special parking spaces. As a result, more and more public buildings, parks, and sidewalks are becoming accessible for those of us who move with crutches or canes or in wheelchairs. But what about private offices and dwellings?

At this time in my life I cannot visit certain friends, or go to certain professional meetings, or even be treated by certain doctors, all for this same reason—stairs. Rectifying the situation would help many people like myself feel that they are fully accredited citizens of our great country.

THE DOOR-HOLDERS: One day my wife and I were on our way into a restaurant that we visit often, because we like the food and it has complete access. I was a little ahead of Gwen, intending to hold the door for her, when a very nice man rushed past us and beat me to this courtesy—but only for my sake, not Gwen's.

I said, "Thank you, but please go ahead. I like to take my time."

"Don't worry," he came back. "I've got plenty of time."

I: "I appreciate your kindness. But I'd really like to open the door myself and hold it for my wife."

He: "This is a heavy door. I'd better hold it for you."

I: "I've opened this door many times. My arms are pretty strong."

He: "That's all right. I'll hold it for you."

I: "You're embarrassing me, my friend."

All I got by way of reply to this was a smile.

As a matter of principle I don't like to yield in arguments

that make me seem more helpless than I am. But at this point there were other people coming up behind us, and I didn't want to create a spectacle. I did resort to one last gesture:

"Precede me, please," I said to my wife. And as we went through in single file, I said to this kind but misinformed man, "Thank you. You're very nice, but please don't do this again."

In another example of this sort I came out of the situation very unhappy with my own response. I was on my way to my office on Madison Avenue. Every morning as I arrived at the entrance to the building where I worked, I would see a certain young man standing at one of the glass doors, waiting for me with the posture of a sergeant at arms. The moment I arrived, his face would break out into a pleased smile. Then he would open the door and stand at attention until I passed through. This little ritual went on day after day. I had no idea who this young man was, and our only verbal communication thus far had been my "thank you."

I was getting more and more embarrassed by this welcome, as it was usually witnessed by people who worked with me. I gave the situation a lot of thought and finally decided I must figure out some way to put a stop to it.

On this particular morning, as I came to the entrance and saw my young man waiting for me at attention, I said something that I will always regret. I said, "My friend, I appreciate all this attention. But my psychiatrist told me I mustn't let other people do things for me that I can do for myself. He said I need the exercise and that too much help is bad for me psychologically."

Having said my piece, I opened one of the other glass doors. As I went through, I got a last glimpse of my private doorman. He looked utterly crestfallen. A pang of remorse lanced through me, and I promised myself that I would apologize to him the next day. I never saw him again.

THE ARM-GRABBERS: One morning, as I was waiting at the curb for the traffic lights to change, a Good Samaritan came up from behind and grabbed my arm to help me. He actually knocked me off balance, but I managed to stay on my feet.

"Thank you," I said when I'd caught my breath; and seeing how concerned he was, I went into my sermonette: "I really appreciate your helpfulness. But may I give you a suggestion? Next time you get that generous impulse to grab a handicapped person's arm, it's best to ask him first if he wants help. He may be enormously grateful to you. But when you take him by surprise, as you've just done with me, you're liable to knock him off his feet. A lot of people like me would rather not be helped. So please, ask first, won't you?"

The same human desire to help prompts many people to grab my arm when I'm getting out of my car, starting up a flight of stairs, or even getting up from a chair in a restaurant. Often as not, rather than brush aside their good intentions, I accept the help. But at other times I stop what I'm doing and ask them, as nicely as I can, to please leave me alone.

THE OVER-SOLICITOUS: Like the arm-grabbers and door-holders, these good people also go out of their way to give you a kind of help you may not need—or want. Just one example:

In the last couple of years, owing to some accidents and surgery, I have been using two crutches instead of one cane. This change in my appearance has given rise to a new kind of exaggerated solicitousness. Whenever I steer my way on a narrow sidewalk, or enter a restaurant or a crowded waiting room or a conference auditorium or the like, people separate like the waters of the Red Sea when Moses led the Jews out of Egypt.

Though I need a clearance of only two feet or so to get myself and my crutches through a crowd, the sight of me coming toward them stirs many people to move way over to the right and left to create a highway for me—about six feet wide, on average.

I know of no way to forestall this kind of courtesy, which puts me in an unwanted spotlight. It makes me feel as if I'm pretending that I'm a visiting dignitary snailing up Fifth Avenue. My usual reaction is to smile and say, "Thank you. I'm really not as wide as I look." Some people respond to that with a pleasant smile; others stare straight ahead and apparently don't respond at all. In any case, I can only hope that my message is getting through.

THE MORTIFIERS: In this category I put all the sincerely helpful people who take it for granted that my sight, my hearing, and my mind are all as impaired as my lower limbs. This includes the thoughtful waitresses and waiters who, when the meal is finished, place the check on the table in front of my wife. I like to reach over and snatch it, but the same waiter or waitress will almost certainly do the same thing again next time we take our table.

Under this same heading come all the people who feel they must address me in a louder-than-normal voice or explain to me what someone else has just said.

This category also includes the cashier in the drugstore who says to my wife as we are exiting, "Tell him to watch out for the step at the door." As if I couldn't hear her or see the step myself!

It includes the nurse who comes to my hospital bed and asks a friend who is visiting me, "Is he going home today?" In this case I can't refrain from telling her, "You can ask *me*, you know. I'm intelligent."

It includes the car salesman who, in my presence, says to my wife, "Why don't you come into my office and let me explain the terms to you?"

Gwen, who knows my feelings, answers, "My husband is the one who's buying the car. Why don't you explain the terms to him?" I flash her a look of gratitude.

THE "EMPATHIZERS": I use the quotation marks to signify that these are the people who tell me how I feel. There's the lovely restaurant hostess who says, "I'll give you a table near the door. I know you don't like to walk."

Another empathizer is the physician who turns to a patient in the waiting room and explains, "I know it's your turn, but I'll take Dr. Oppenheim first, because he's disabled and it's a hardship for him to wait. I'm sure you won't mind."

Naturally, the very nice patient nods and says, "No problem."

I would like to ask the doctor not to embarrass me by leaping to such an unwarranted conclusion. Instead I protest that I don't want to take somebody else's turn on the grounds of disability. "I'd rather wait my turn," I say.

But the doctor is in no mood for argument, and of course I don't want to make a scene. I turn to the patient I'm displacing and say, "That's very kind of you. I hope you don't mind." Again he professes not to mind at all.

I know this physician and like him very much. But I'm afraid I'm not getting my message across to him.

More or less in this same category of "empathizers" is a patient of mine who professed to be a healer and offered to cure my pain. I told her that I wasn't in any pain, which happened to be true, and politely declined. She was a little taken aback because, as she put it, "I can tell that you're in pain."

THE THOUGHTLESS: These are the people who will say things without any consciousness of the unhappy effect their words might have on a handicapped person. Conspicuous in this category are some members of the medical profession, especially—though I hesitate to generalize— surgeons.

During my postoperative recovery at one of America's greatest hospitals, the orthopedist who had implanted a partial hip replacement in me was discussing his procedure with a resident at my bedside. The surgeon, who is considered one of the best in his field, pulled my sheet back and told me to turn over. The resident, who never introduced himself, ran his finger along the incision.

Turning to the surgeon, the resident asked, "How come you made such a crooked incision?"

The surgeon gave him what I thought was a rather lame technical reply. The incident seems trivial, but its immediate effect on me was to generate a depressing question in my mind: Had this highly respected surgeon done a botch job on me?

While I was still debating on how to handle this insulting behavior, the surgeon pulled the sheet back over me and the two of them strode out.

Another candidate for inclusion in the thoughtless category is a certain orthotist or bracemaker. While discussing some modifications to my brace, he kept talking about accommodating to my "deformity."

Words like that are powerful. They evoke images. The word "deformity" suggests a hideous, twisted body part. When I was younger and still coping with my own body image, that word would have triggered a long-lasting depression in me. Now I feel it reflects on the person who uses it so insensitively.

In the same category is the orthopedic specialist who told a patient I know, "You'll never use that arm again." I would like to say to this doctor that in the medical vocabulary "never" is a dirty word. There are always exceptions to such predictions. Moreover, there are constant advances in medicine that may prove the doctor wrong. So why demoralize a patient with such a grim but shaky prediction?

An orthopedist I once consulted for pain in my hands expressed grave concern, which I believe was sincere. He diagnosed the carpel tunnel syndrome and told me that in six months my fingers would be bent like claws, unable to straighten out, unless I had prompt surgery. When I expressed doubt, he sent me to a specialist who examined my hands with a computerized machine. She confirmed the first doctor's diagnosis and said the operation was a must.

I went to still another orthopedist. He suggested that arm splints worn at night might spare me from this surgery. Six months later my hands were perfectly normal.

Finally I must include in this category a friend of mine who broke a leg in a skiing accident. "Now I know how *you* feel," he told me.

I didn't disillusion him, but I'm sure he had no idea how I feel. His handicap was temporary; he could look forward to being cured and resuming all his normal activities in a few weeks. He didn't have to develop all sorts of coping techniques. He didn't realize that having a permanent disability is something entirely different. He will never have to go through the pangs of feeling isolated because of his appearance.

On the other side of the ledger, he may never know the rewards my handicap has brought me.

THE VIOLATORS: The people I am about to describe are—well, I have some difficulty putting them in the category of "angels," but I will try to be charitable. They are the able-bodied drivers who have no hesitation about pulling into a parking place reserved for the handicapped. When reminded by my wife or me that this not only may subject the driver to a fine, but, more important, may create a hardship for some person who needs the space, they have quite a variety of responses. Here is a selection:

A healthy-looking young woman: "I have a weak heart." When asked why she doesn't have a handicapped license, she answers, "They told me it's in the mail." And off she runs.

A violator in the parking lot of a restaurant: "I'll only be a few minutes." And into the restaurant he goes with a woman and a child.

A man parked his Cadillac in a handicapped space in front of an office building: When I try to speak to him, he ignores me and walks into the building. A woman comes over and tells me, "He's the company president. He parks there every day—the jerk!"

The driver of a delivery van who is unloading packages on a narrow street in front of a building I need to enter: "I'll be finished in a couple of minutes." I tell him I can't wait while I'm double-parked, because I'm holding up traffic. In response, he picks up one of the packages on the street and carries it into the building.

A young male in a red sports car at the license bureau's parking lot: "Oh, there'll be plenty of other spaces!"

The chauffeur of an elongated limousine in downtown Manhattan: "My boss had to go to the bathroom."

A variant of the parking hog is the person who makes a handicapped space useless. A very common example of this is to be found in supermarket parking lots. Thoughtless men and women frequently leave their shopping carts in the spaces reserved for the handicapped, creating a hardship for the person on crutches.

When I see one of these violators getting into his car, I try to talk to him (or her). A frequent response is that he jumps into his car and drives off. A less frequent response is that the violator says, "I'm sorry," and moves the cart out of the way. In most cases, however, the shopper is gone by the time I reach the scene.

Winter weather brings another kind of space spoiler. One recent morning, my wife and I drove to the local post office, only to find the one space reserved for the handicapped was occupied by a pile of snow that had been shoveled into it. A post-office employee was still busy enlarging the pile. The only space available was at the far end of the lot and would have entailed a long, slippery walk for me.

My wife jumped out of the car and reminded the man that he was disregarding the needs of the people for whom the space was reserved.

His answer: "Oh, this space doesn't get a lot of use."

Gwen marched right off and into the office of the acting postmaster, where she indignantly reported the offense.

Said he: "Don't worry. I promise you that it'll be cleared by noon." It wasn't. The space remained blocked until the day the snow melted.

I am happy to report that police officers are now being assigned to parking lots in New York's malls for the specific purpose of ticketing these violators.

———————

TO RELATIVES, FRIENDS, AND STRANGERS: Are there any occasions when you should override a handicapped person if he persistently declines to accept your help? My answer to that would be Yes, but not often. For instance, in the situation described above, Amy, our guest, saw me carrying her suitcase to the car, so she knew I could do it. But if she had seen me stumble and skin my knee, her training as a nurse would rightly have led her to think that she knew better than I. In such a case, she might have chosen to hurt my feelings in order to protect me from further harm.

When you know that a handicapped person is being foolhardy, would you be justified in helping him in spite of his protests, or is it better to respect his feelings? The question is certainly a sticky one, and I wouldn't presume to give advice sight unseen. Each instance is different, and you must find your own answer. In any event, you have shown your concern by asking him, and I hope that he responds with an expression of gratitude.

To get up in the middle of the night to carry your suitcase to the car, knowing very well how he felt and what he could do—that, I think, is bringing a kind impulse to an ignoble end.

My suggestion: Ask first if he wants the help. If he doesn't, respect his wishes. But if you feel you know better than he what the dangers are, discuss the situation with him instead of taking matters into your own hands. If, after all this, you still override him, you will know that you are hurting his feelings. He may then be angry at you, but who is to say that either of your judgments is right?

TO ALL PEOPLE WITH A GENUINE DESIRE TO HELP: It is heartening to know that there are so many wonderfully kind people like yourself in this harsh world. Since your desire to be helpful is sincere, I can only hope that you do not take any of the above paragraphs as put-downs. I can assure you that your kindness is fully appreciated and that any misconceptions about the handicapped that you may have acquired from popular stereotypes are well understood.

It is precisely because I know of your real desire to be helpful that I am offering you this compendium of do's and don'ts so that you may sharpen your skills—not only in understanding the handicapped but in empathizing with all kinds of people who may be different from yourself.

One thing to keep in mind when you want to help a handicapped person is that most people who are coping with an impaired body could tell you that the last thing they want is pity. While you are piloting a polio victim across a street and your heart is going out to him, please avoid such remarks as, "I know how difficult your life must be!" Unless your helpee is a person of enormous understanding, he may want to turn around and bite you.

Next time you have a reflex impulse to help a disabled person, won't you pause for a second to think about it and then offer your assistance in an enlightened way?

————

TO THE HANDICAPPED: After reading the above examples, you may get the impression that I sometimes reacted with uncalled-for tartness to gestures of kindness and helpfulness. And you'd be right. In my younger days I was so sensitive about my handicap that I would flare up when people treated me as if I were more helpless than I actually was. When a Good Samaritan grabbed my arm without asking me, my internal reaction was to say, "Get the hell away from me!" I'm afraid it was part of the same self-protective arrogance that I displayed all through my childhood and youth.

But there were times when I had to swallow my arrogance and accept assistance. Little by little these occasions helped me to realize that whenever another human being spontaneously reached out to me, I should be thankful that there are so many good people who are ready to help. Today, there are some occasions when I even accept help that I truly don't need so that I can give a nice person the feeling that he has done his good deed for the day.

A point to remember: No matter how self-sufficient you would like to be, there are those times when you really do need help. Don't be ashamed, as I once was, to ask for it. You and the person who responds to your honest request will both feel good about it.

And when some kind person insists on holding the door for you, and you would rather hold it yourself to show your wife a courtesy, try not to get angry or feel bad about yourself. A good strategy is simply to accept his kindness and thank him. But then say to your wife, "After you, my dear." That way you may be sending him an acceptable message.

EPILOGUE

As I look back on my life, I am awed and grateful for the way my Creator has put opportunities in my path right at the appropriate moment to help me through each of my difficulties. These include troubled parents, a somewhat messed-up childhood, social isolation at schools, a shame-filled body image, and some major physical ailments besides polio, along with an "invariably fatal" cancer (I sure beat the odds on that one!). All these troubles have turned out to be challenges, and, if I should die tomorrow, I know that I can look back with satisfaction on a life of growth and service.

I believe that I can say now, without blushing, that polio has given me the inner fiber to face life with a sense of adventure and joy. It has led me out of pits of fear and despair to the deepest kind of happiness and fulfillment through work and love.

More than that: It has brought me full circle back to that little boy watching the sunrise from a wheelchair.

ABOUT THE AUTHOR

Garrett Oppenheim is the founder and director of Confide—Personal Counseling Services in Tappan, New York. He holds board certifications as a medical psychotherapist, a hypnotherapist, a sex therapist, and a counselor. He is most widely known for his pioneering work in past-life therapy.

He is the author of more than 100 articles that have appeared in professional and popular periodicals, and his work in hypnotherapy has been featured in Time-Life books and numerous newspapers and magazines.

Prior to his career in personal counseling, Dr. Oppenheim was a journalist with the nation's leading newspapers, including the *Wall Street Journal* and the *New York Times.*

He received his doctor of philosophy degree from Columbia Pacific University.

What Is A.R.E.?

The Association for Research and Enlightenment, Inc. (A.R.E.®), is the international headquarters for the work of Edgar Cayce (1877-1945), who is considered the best-documented psychic of the twentieth century. Founded in 1931, the A.R.E. consists of a community of people from all walks of life and spiritual traditions, who have found meaningful and life-transformative insights from the readings of Edgar Cayce.

Although A.R.E. headquarters is located in Virginia Beach, Virginia—where visitors are always welcome—the A.R.E. community is a global network of individuals who offer conferences, educational activities, and fellowship around the world. People of every age are invited to participate in programs that focus on such topics as holistic health, dreams, reincarnation, ESP, the power of the mind, meditation, and personal spirituality.

In addition to study groups and various activities, the A.R.E. offers membership benefits and services, a bimonthly magazine, a newsletter, extracts from the Cayce readings, conferences, international tours, a massage school curriculum, an impressive volunteer network, a retreat-type camp for children and adults, and A.R.E. contacts around the world. A.R.E. also maintains an affiliation with Atlantic University, which offers a master's degree program in Transpersonal Studies.

For additional information about A.R.E. activities hosted near you, please contact:

A.R.E.
67th St. and Atlantic Ave.
P.O. Box 595
Virginia Beach, VA 23451-0595
(804) 428-3588

A.R.E. Press

A.R.E. Press is a publisher and distributor of books, audiotapes, and videos that offer guidance for a more fulfilling life. Our products are based on, or are compatible with, the concepts in the psychic readings of Edgar Cayce.

We especially seek to create products which carry forward the inspirational story of individuals who have made practical application of the Cayce legacy.

For a free catalog, please write to A.R.E. Press at the address below or call toll free 1-800-723-1112. For any other information, please call 804-428-3588.

A.R.E. Press
Sixty-Eighth & Atlantic Avenue
P.O. Box 656
Virginia Beach, VA 23451-0656